# treatment kind and fair

## letters to a young doctor

# Perri Klass, M.D.

## treatment kind and fair

### letters to a young doctor

BASIC
BOOKS

A Member of the Perseus Books Group
New York

Copyright © 2007 by Perri Klass, M. D.

Published by Basic Books, A Member of the Perseus Books Group

Books published by Basic Books are available at special discounts for bulk purchases in the United States by corporations, institutions, and other organizations. For more information, please contact the Special Markets Department at the Perseus Books Group, 2300 Chestnut Street, Suite 200, Philadelphia, PA 19103, or call (800) 810-4145, extension 5000, or e-mail special.markets@perseusbooks.com.

Library of Congress Cataloging-in-Publication Data

Klass, Perri, 1958–
    Treatment kind and fair : letters to a young doctor / Perri Klass.
        p. ; cm.
    HC ISBN: 978-0-465-03777-3
    PB ISBN: 978-0-465-03778-0  1. Medicine—Vocational guidance. 2. Physicians—Attitudes. 3. Physician and patient. I. Title.
    [DNLM: 1. Physician's Role. 2. Career Choice. 3. Physician-Patient Relations. W 62 K63t 2007]

R690.K62 2007

610.69—dc22

2007006848


10  9  8  7  6  5  4  3  2  1

For Benjamin Orlando Klass, in so many ways—
born to a medical student, practical pediatric tutor
throughout residency, and source of endless and
continuing delight,
—*With love.*

*Two and twenty now he's rising,*
*And alone he's fit to fly,*
*Which we're bent on signalizing*
*With unusual revelry.*
*Here's good luck to Frederic's ventures!*
*Frederic's out of his indentures.*

—W. S. Gilbert, *The Pirates of Penzance*

# ▨ Contents

# ■ Preface

Medicine is not exactly an underexposed profession. There are white-coated doctors on every news show, reassuring you or scaring you about bird flu or HIV or SARS, solemnly explaining new scientific miracles or celebrity illnesses, or perhaps just making you feel guilty about what you eat. In the bookstore you will find medical thrillers (Killer viruses! Sinister trading in human organs!) and medical memoirs (the dehumanizing grind of medical school, the overworked hell of residency). There are whole nests of gorgeous young doctors out there on television dramas, saving lives and falling into bed with one another, and there are gruff senior doctors grilling them and putting them through hell (for their own good) and occasionally falling into bed with them (how can they help it, everyone is so gorgeous).

If you are thinking about medicine as a career, most colleges offer a vast machinery of premed counseling and advising, with special offices and regular meetings to help you navigate the elaborate process of making yourself into a medical student. Now there are Web sites

where you can track every tiny step in the drill of applying to medical school, and trade minute details about
which interviewer at which school asked which tough
questions. I know this because my own son, Orlando,
who was born back when I was in medical school, is now
on this same path. Hanging over his shoulder, I have
been introduced to the wonderful world of online medical school applications and premed chat rooms, as well
as Web sites with names like studentdoctor.net and as-
piringdocs.org where you can calculate your chances of
admission or read about the triumphs and humiliations
of your competitors.

Orlando is the representative "young doctor" to
whom I am addressing these letters; I am proud and delighted that he has chosen medicine, and as a parent, I
want to guide him away from my mistakes and help him
find the joy and passion and complexity that I believe
this profession can offer. But like the rest of you who are
reading this book, my son is no fool—this writing about
medicine will only be useful if I'm honest about the
problems and the headaches.

I've been writing about medicine ever since I was a
young doctor myself—actually, ever since I was a medical student. In my first year of medical school, back in
1982, I started writing about my training and the process
of turning people into doctors. My goal was to offer a
window into this endlessly interesting new medical
world that was just opening up to me. It turned out that

there were readers—and not just medical people—who were interested in a behind-the-scenes look at the profession I was joining. They wanted to understand how doctors became fluent in the jargon I was learning to speak or to follow along as I tried to dissect the macho-tinged rivalries among different teams of doctors caring for the same patient.

As I was starting medical school, people gave me books about medical education. I read only a couple, but they seemed to me out-of-date, frequently whiny, and often pompous. So I ended up writing my own book from my own perspective as a woman going to medical school in the 1980s. The book was called *A Not Entirely Benign Procedure*, and in it I tried not to take myself too seriously and not to take medicine too seriously. I continued writing about my training all through my pediatric residency, so I ended up with a book about residency as well.

Let me be honest: I did not love medical school. I did not always understand why I was doing what I was doing, and I did not always like what was happening to me. As I look back, I understand that I was not always well taught, but I also understand that I failed to take full advantage of all the chances to learn. Now that I have been practicing for well over a decade, now that I try hard to study around the busy edges of my life, I sometimes feel irritated with my arrogant younger self: *Why didn't you understand the importance of what you were learning? Why didn't you take more trouble to understand?* On the other hand, I loved residency—loved working with children, loved the hospital, loved the excitement of really being a doctor. I was chronically miserable and sleep-deprived (or chronically miserable *because* I was sleep-deprived), but I was also exhilarated. Those three years were a strange mix of adrenaline and exhaustion. And I managed to keep writing.

My life in medicine has involved a mix—I practiced primary-care pediatrics in a health center in Boston for more than a decade, taking care of an interesting population of urban children. At the same time, I had an academic appointment at Boston University School of Medicine, where I did some pediatric infectious diseases work, including a good deal of travel medicine (helping people stay healthy while they travel and doing assessments of new immigrants and refugees). At the same time, I have been heavily involved with a program called Reach Out and Read, which works through pediatricians and family doctors and nurses who take care of children to promote reading aloud and early literacy. So my life was a mix of seeing patients and of on-call evenings answering phone calls from parents, and then some hospital-based subspecialty work and advocacy work in the nonprofit world. Most academic doctors end up with a pieced-together life of this kind, following their interests, following patient-care needs, changing over time. Now I work at New York University, seeing patients and supervising residents in the clinic at Bellevue, again an inner-city primary-care population. I also teach in NYU's journalism department because I have kept on writing.

Writing about medicine and medical training and medical practice has always added grace notes to my life in medicine. The training is crowded and intense, and for most doctors, the daily clinical practice is also crowded and intense. Characters and plots and subplots and dialogue and incidents and responsibility fill the hours, because your job takes you into people's lives and into their families and into their minds and their sorrows. When I write about medicine, I write about patients, always trying to pin down the complicated pieces of other people's lives that go spinning past me. As a resident, exhausted beyond belief, I would come home and sit down and write the story of a surprising patient encounter, a hospital moment that I felt I would never forget. A month or two later I would look at the reference and the child would have slipped my mind completely, displaced by the parade of children and families and conversations and exam-room encounters and unfolding medical histories. I think that ever since those residency days, I have been trying to do two different things by keeping track of my patients and noting down some of their stories. First, I have been trying to hold on to those moments of remarkable contact with children and families. I know they blur and disappear, and I don't want to lose them, or to forget the lessons they teach. Second, I have been trying to see myself clearly, to track my own changing professional persona.

Medicine offers many learning opportunities designed to last you your whole life long, but it is not, by and large, a reflective profession. Writing about medicine has always offered me a way to watch my own evolution, to try to understand the changes that medical training and medical practice can bring about. I've enjoyed writing about my patients and about my colleagues, and I've enjoyed writing about myself. This book, though, is different. This is a chance to write directly to someone considering medicine as a profession—or starting out in medicine as a profession—and by great good fortune, I was writing this book just as my oldest child was applying to medical school. So whenever I tried to picture that "young doctor" to whom I was writing, it was my son's face that swam into view. Writing this book has given me a chance to dispense a combination of maternal and medical wisdom.

In fact, I realize I feel somewhat maternal toward all young people who are considering devoting their lives to medicine. They remind me of myself and of my friends and my classmates—but they also inspire me with awe and envy. I am impressed by their willingness to work, and their willingness to take on the increasingly overwhelming flood of medical research and medical information. I am delighted to see that they understand the appeal of this profession despite the constant flow of news articles on the economic and administrative and ethical quagmires in which doctors today supposedly find themselves struggling. And I envy them the choices they have—the opportunity to survey the complex and rich field of medicine and find their own personal places. I would save them from all my mistakes and bad choices if I could, but they need to find their own mistakes. I would like to tell them—my son and all the others—a little bit about this compelling world, which I think remains mysterious, despite all the memoirs and all the television shows. (By the way, most young doctors aren't as gorgeous as all that, and there is considerably less sex in your average residency program than in your average prime-time TV show—but you knew that already, didn't you?) I would like to help my readers understand what it feels like to be a doctor—to do the everyday job of it—and how they will change and develop so they will be ready to do that everyday job.

Let me say a word about the title of the book. It comes from a poem by Hillaire Belloc, and the poem is about, of all things, being kind to frogs. But the phrase "a treatment kind and fair" seemed to evoke exactly what we hope, as doctors, to provide for our patients. Beyond that, it suggested something else to me as I thought about my son and other smart young people going into medicine: I want the field itself to treat you kindly and to treat you fairly. Medicine will exact from you all kinds of dedication and professional obligations—and I want you to be well treated in return.

The letters in this book roughly parallel medical training, though I promise to digress in all directions. The first part focuses on medical school, on getting in and learning the basic skills—like how to examine a patient—that define the medical profession. The second part takes on a range of topics that come to the fore during residency, as you find and hold your own place in medicine, keep track of the information and the science that you need to do your job, and learn to cope with the uncertainty of your choices and the certainty of wrong decisions and outright mistakes. The final section is mostly about practicing medicine: taking care of patients, listening to their stories and their secrets, caring for people as they die, and integrating all of this into your life.

"People will always need doctors" was the once-upon-a-time clichéd advice of the once-upon-a-time clichéd mother, pushing a child in the direction of a safe and sure career. But I say it to you now not to urge you toward security. I say it to you because I have come to believe that it is profoundly true—people will always need doctors, and by entering this profession, you will grapple with uncertainty and insecurity, with tragedy and pain, and above all, you will meet people's needs. This is a good job and an honorable job, and an endlessly interesting job. But it's not a simple job, and we've got a lot to talk about.

# 1

■ Deciding to Be a Doctor—
Choosing and Being Chosen, and
Making Your Mother Proud

*A twenty-two-year-old male presents with anxiety and disturbed sleep. He has previously been in good health, and has recently applied to twenty medical schools. He describes an inability to stay away from his e-mail, where he is obsessively checking for responses, indications that his application files are complete, and interview invitations. He is drinking six to seven cups of coffee a day. When he does fall asleep, he dreams about kindly figures in white coats with stethoscopes bending over him and listening to his heart.*

*Dear Orlando,*

So you're really going to do it! You have to give me credit—I may be your mother, but you have to admit, I haven't pushed you to be a doctor. It was a real matter of principle with me—first that you should choose work that really drew you, and second, that however much I love medicine for myself, there would be something wrong with pressuring you to follow the same path. But you've been saying ever since high school that you thought you wanted to go to medical school, and now here we are, and you're actually applying, and I have a confession to make: I'm totally delighted. And now I can admit several things that I haven't quite let myself say: I think it's a wonderful choice, I think medicine will let you exercise and extend all your skills and talents, I think you'll mostly enjoy the training process (well, I think you'll hate some of it, but I think you'll kind of enjoy hating it, and I'll explain what I mean by that a little later on), and I think you'll find yourself with a fascinating set of intellectual challenges and choices, and a busy and rewarding professional life. I think medicine will make good use of you, and you will make good use of medicine.

And I guess I'm a little flattered. You may not mean it this way at all—you may look on me as a member of a completely different species—but I can't help feeling that your decision to go to medical school must mean that you look at your own childhood and feel I did an okay job. You, after all, are my medical school baby. I got pregnant during my first year of medical school, and you were born in January of my second year. You were one and a half when we went to London so I could study for a month at the London School of Tropical Medicine and

Hygiene—wonderful leprosy clinics, by the way, I highly recommend them! You turned two in New Delhi, where I was spending a month as a visiting medical student at the All India Institute of Medicine. And you were two and a half when I started my pediatric residency at Boston Children's Hospital, and five and a half when I finished it. In the early 1990s I went on to do a fellowship in pediatric infectious diseases, and I spent a significant part of my professional life then dealing with children infected with HIV, because that was when the demographics of the AIDS epidemic began to shift in the United States, with more women infected and bearing infected babies.

During all those residency and fellowship years, you were my home model of a healthy child. Every time someone asked a question about development—at what age should a child sit up alone, start to walk, speak in full sentences—I quickly thought about you. You were also my greatest delight, and since I was working those insane residency hours, I spent a lot of time missing you.

I know you remember there were nights during those years when your father used to bring you to visit in the hospital—we would eat together in the cafeteria. And you made your theatrical debut in the holiday show put on by my group of Children's Hospital interns and residents. There was a skit about the emergency room, and an intern's dread of seeing yet another incredibly complex, incredibly sick pediatric patient. His lines went something like this: "It's probably a child with multiple congenital anomalies on seventeen medications I've never heard of, with a compromised airway and a weakened immune system coming in with a fever of unknown origin—and I've already had six of those tonight!" And at that point, the four-year-old you popped out from under a chair, pointing to your ear and complaining that it hurt. And the intern realized that in fact her next patient was a kid with an ear infection—at which point a heavenly choir sang a version of the "Hallelujah Chorus," with lyrics like "Hallelujah! Hallelujah! This child has got otitis!" Believe me, until you've heard a chorus of residents squeezing in all the syllables of various antibiotics, all more or less to the tune of Handel, you haven't lived (Hallelujah! Hallelujah! We will give him amoxicillin! Cephalosporins!). Don't worry, you will get to take part in many such shows; they are an absolute staple of medical education. Your youthful theatrical promise is about to be realized. But you will never again be as cute as you were when you popped out from under that chair.

Your early childhood was shaped by the processes and imperatives of medical training, and your whole life after that was affected by my schedule and my on-call rotations and my preoccupations and anxieties. In my darker moments, I sometimes imagined a child telling me that it had been a rotten way to grow up. So there is a certain thrill, and even a feeling of redemption, in having that child declare his intention of building a similar life for himself.

Okay, now you have to build that life. You understand that this is a long training, you're going to apply to medical school, arduous all by itself. Then you're going to do your four years of medical school, and after that your residency—mine was three years, in pediatrics; if you stay with the idea of doing surgery, yours could be anywhere from five to seven years. And then a fellowship if you want to do one—another three years or so of training and research in a subspecialty. This is how you are going to spend your twenties and probably your early thirties. Recently, I met a young woman who was finishing medical school and was applying for a residency at the hospital where I work. She said something that I liked very much. She said her decision to go into medicine had come about in part because she so liked being a student, and she wanted to find a career where she would be a student for her whole life. Medicine will give you that, and I hope you will enjoy it. You will be a student and a teacher.

So what I'm going to do now is tell you how I have spent my own life as a student. I'm going to tell you what it's like learning to take care of patients—to listen to their stories and to touch their bodies. I'm going to tell you about the challenge of keeping up with science as new discoveries are made, and about the complexities of making a living as a doctor as medicine changes. I'm going to tell you why it's fun for me to get up in the morning and go to work—and sometimes why it's hard for me to fall asleep at night, because I'm worrying, or beating myself up. I'm going to tell you about the choices I've made within medicine, but also about some of the ones I wish I'd had the chance to make—and about all the others that are open to you.

•

Once upon a time, there was a belief that people went into medicine in order to make a good living—well, okay, to get rich. They would be rich doctors whose wives wore mink coats, who played golf on fancy country clubs. I remember a humorous novel called *The Serial* about upscale life in Marin County, near San Francisco, in the 1970s. In one scene the protagonist, a guy who works in a bank, finds himself taking a woman to a fancy French restaurant, and he realizes, to his distress, that the parking lot is full of luxury cars with MD license plates, which immediately tells him he's way out of his price range. Sure enough, the restaurant is full of doctors, and our hero is thoroughly humiliated; he has to pretend to have a sudden attack of back pain and beat a hasty retreat.

I don't think that scene would play well today. Doctors earn perfectly respectable incomes, but if you meet anyone who's going into this field because it's where the money is—well, how can I say this?—I would not trust that person to make a diagnosis involving native intelligence, efficient fact-finding, or basic good sense. I promise you that many of your college classmates are going to be getting rich on Wall Street or in corporate law or business, while you are working eighty hours a week as a resident, earning something that comes out perilously near the minimum wage when you calculate it on an hourly basis.

That doesn't mean I'm whining, and neither should you. Doctors are definitely not poor. What medicine *does* offer, in the making-a-living category, is a chance to earn a respectable income doing the thing that you will have trained to do. If you train as a doctor, you will work as a doctor, and that is no small thing. But the much bigger, grander thing is that medicine will offer you a chance to earn that respectable income by doing something genuinely interesting and genuinely rewarding every single day of your working life, by staying in touch with science and technology, and by getting in touch with the lives of other people.

You are struggling right now with your medical school application essays, and I know that it can be hard to find a new way of saying all these things: *I want to help people* (please, whatever you do, don't say that; when I worked as a premed adviser, I spent much of my time crossing it out of students' essays. Yeah, yeah, we know, you want to help people—now tell us something we don't know!). *I want to combine my interest in science with my desire to help people* (what did I tell you about saying you want to help people!). *I think medicine will be a very rewarding career* (yeah, you and everybody else—and let me guess, it will be rewarding because you'll get to help people, right?). On the other hand, all of these things are perfectly true: medicine *will* put you in a position to spend your professional life helping people, and that *is* profoundly rewarding.

When I was a first-year medical student, we were matched up with clinical tutors. Each group of four medical students would meet with a doctor who was supposed to take us into the hospital and show us a little real medicine. My tutor was a pediatric intensivist. She worked in the pediatric intensive care unit, with the sickest kids in the hospital. Horrendous trauma, overwhelming bacterial infections, life-threatening respiratory distress—to get into the PICU, a child had to be so seriously sick that almost half of those who were admitted didn't make it out. That's unusual in pediatrics—a 50 percent mortality rate—and it's grueling. Even the mortality rate in pediatric oncology is down around 10 percent. Nobody ever gets used to seeing children die. But I still remember the day our tutor told us a harrowing story of a healthy, happy girl who had contracted toxic shock syndrome and had come close to dying. She had needed massive technological supports for her heart, her blood pressure, her lungs. Listening to the doctor describe it, we got the sense of a personal battle that the intensive care unit staff had fought, hour by hour, body system by body system, to keep this child alive, while they waited for the antibiotics to turn the infection around.

And they had won. The girl had turned the corner, she had come through, our tutor told us as we made our way to the girl's hospital room. And now—our tutor threw open the door with a flourish and announced, "*This* is the glory of pediatrics!" And there she was: a kid, sitting up in her hospital bed, laughing and being silly with her parents. And that is the glory of pediatrics: that children, when they recover, go back to being children, that they are as resilient as they are, that when you win a battle like this, you win it for decades and decades of healthy life. My tutor didn't actually say to us—worshipful, awestruck first-year medical students that we were— tell me why anyone would do any other job than this, but we understood it. And we also understood that her sense of pride and sense of victory were rooted in the reality of other battles lost and other pediatric bedsides where there had been no laughter and jubilation.

What a good and interesting job you're choosing! It's a job that in the larger sense touches every human being—we all go through this world in bodies, and we are all literally and figuratively touched at so many points by illness and by the medical profession. Doctors are engaged with individual humans at the level that makes everyone human.

•

I don't know if you can understand—I don't know if anyone your age can understand—how thrilling it is to see you make this choice. When I interview intern applicants, every time I talk to one who is smart and tough and idealistic (and most of them are smart and tough and idealistic), I feel a sharp sense of joy that this young person is going into pediatrics. And I feel a broader, deeper sense of pride that medicine as a profession continues to exercise its pull.

But there's something else as well—there's the mom thing, the woman thing, the family-and-career thing. It's not my favorite subject, but it needs to be talked about. In 1982, when I started medical school, the entering class was about 30 percent female. And that felt good; I didn't feel like the only woman in the room. I didn't feel that I had to get everything right, or that I had to be one of the best students. No, I felt I was part of a strong female presence. I can remember paging through old medical school yearbooks, though, yearbooks from only fifteen or twenty years earlier, and seeing page after page after page of clean-cut young white male faces, and thinking dizzily about how quickly medicine had changed.

Your medical school class will be fifty-fifty (with both the men and the women significantly more varied by race and ethnicity than they were in my era)—and that means that you will be in a profession, overall, that will be fifty-fifty. Not necessarily every subset—there's plenty of variation from urology to psychiatry to cardiothoracic surgery to ob-gyn—but fifty-fifty overall. That is remarkable. Yes, I could lecture you about the need to promote more women to positions of authority, the need for more female department chairs, the need to encourage women to go into the surgical subspecialties in greater numbers. But we should also celebrate the reality that a female medical student is now just a medical student, a female doctor is just a doctor.

In the late 1980s, I wrote a story for the *New York Times Magazine* about the greater number of women going into medicine, which they published under the title "Are Women Better Doctors?" I didn't think it was the best title. Yes, I had asked the women doctors I interviewed whether they thought there were differences in how men and women practiced medicine, and yes, the women had essentially all said, yes, there are differences, let's face it, we're better! But I meant to include this half-humorously, more as evidence of woman-doctor pride and solidarity than anything else. The story ran with that title, and I got dozens and dozens of angry letters, mostly from doctors, male and female, all objecting to the title rather than to the article. The question itself was offensive, they said. A good doctor is a good doctor; there are bad female doctors and good male doctors and vice versa. How would you like it, several of the letters queried, if you saw an article published with a title like, are men better doctors, are whites better doctors, are Jews better doctors?

And they weren't wrong—it was an offensive formulation—though I also remember thinking at the time that it would be good if we could all lighten up a little. I was reminded of an incident in medical school when the admissions office began to object that the women's medical student organization was making special efforts to host visiting female applicants, and the minority students' association was hosting minority applicants, and so on—and it wasn't fair, the admissions officers complained, because no one was specially hosting the white men. There was a pause and then someone said, wow, so do you think there'll be any of them in next year's class?

I closed that *New York Times* article with a story about you—I think you were three or four at the time. It was about the time I told you that you were going to see your new pediatrician, and you looked at me nervously and said, "Is she a nice doctor?" I realized that because you knew me and my friends, you took for granted that all doctors were women, and I needed to prepare you to see your male pediatrician. So I told you, gently but (I hope) encouragingly, that boys could be doctors, too. And look at you now!

Speaking of women doctors, do you remember that particular advice I gave you about medical school interviews? If you're interviewed by a woman faculty member, I said, be especially sure to emphasize not just that you're the child of a physician—tell them explicitly that your *mother* is a doctor. They'll really like that. And you looked at me a bit blankly and said, "Why do you say that?" And I was completely charmed that you didn't know why, but all I said was, "It's a long story, dear. Lots of history. Just trust me on this one."

So yes, let's talk about getting in. As you know very well, after four years of undergraduate premed work, this is not set up to be easy. The medical profession regulates the number of medical schools, and the number of places available in each medical school, and they keep the lid on tight. That's why plenty of qualified undergraduates still end up going overseas for their medical training; there aren't enough spots available in the 125 accredited U.S. medical schools. In fact, U.S. medical schools don't graduate nearly enough doctors every year to fill the accredited U.S. residency programs, which is why so many need to fill their slots with foreign medical school graduates. That's why I can tell you so confidently: If you train as a doctor in the United States, you will be able to work as a doctor in the United States.

But that also means that getting into medical school becomes the giant hurdle. If you get in, then medical school will teach you enough to pass the licensing exam, and you will find a residency spot. You aren't guaranteed the spot you want, or even the specialty you want. Some fields like dermatology and ophthalmology and certain surgical subspecialties have comparatively few spots and way too many applicants, but unless you are a complete and total screwup (and even then, in many cases), you will end up with a residency and a license and a job as a physician. It isn't like law: If you're willing to go far enough down the hierarchy of law schools, there's a school somewhere that will accept you. There is no limit set on the number of lawyers trained. On the other hand, a law degree guarantees you nothing in the way of a job. Lawyers are regulated by supply and demand. Not so doctors. No matter the demand, the domestic supply is limited to those 125 medical schools, and their small classes. Other doctors have to come in from overseas, pass additional (and formidable) licensing exams, and sometimes do major pieces of their training all over again.

So yes, getting one of those spots in one of those small classes at those medical schools is still a big deal. At least half of medical school applicants don't find a place in the United States—and remember, these are all students who have managed to complete (and presumably pass) the premed courses. They've invested a considerable amount of effort and energy and intellectual capital and sweat, since the premed courses themselves were set up to be stumbling blocks, or opportunities for serious weeding out. But medical school itself, once you're in, is not a weeding-out kind of experience. There used to be a legend at Harvard Law School about a professor saying to the students on day one of year one, look to your right, look to your left—one of you three will be gone by the end of the year. The medical school equivalent would be, look to your right, look to your left, we will do whatever it takes to make all three of you into doctors. A medical school has a tremendous sense of investment in every student in the (relatively small) entering class; they are all supposed to make it through and pass their boards and earn their MD degrees and find themselves reciting the Hippocratic Oath.

For this reason, it's an elaborate and lengthy admissions process. And I have to admit to you that when I think about these admissions committees considering you, Orlando, I have a motherly wish to admonish you in all kinds of traditional ways: Wear a suit! Shine your shoes! Stand up when someone comes into the room! Call your interviewers Sir or Ma'am or Doctor, shake hands firmly, look 'em in the eye!

I focus on the interview because it is so important for medical school. Each medical school interviews only a certain number of applicants for every spot, and they won't bother interviewing people they don't think have a reasonable chance of being admitted. So getting an interview is something of a triumph all by itself. Back in the old days, medical school interviews were legendary. Everybody knew a story about a stress interview, an outrageous interview, a completely unfair out-of-left-field interview. The student who is asked to open the window, and it's nailed shut. Or the student who is grilled at length on the small technical details of the economics of health care in America today, and is never asked a single why-do-you-want-to-be-a-doctor

question. You're unlikely to have a stress interview—
even in my day they were more legend than reality. But
you better be ready for those regular old non-stress interviews. In addition to your well-polished shoes and
manners, be sure you read the newspaper carefully
every day, looking for health stories, and be sure you
have an opinion you've thought out on the big medical
controversies of the day. For that matter, be sure you
have an opinion on what is the biggest problem facing
American medicine today; that's an easy all-purpose
question for any interviewer who hasn't read your file
closely.

Above all, think about how you can convey how
much you want to do this. They are looking for people
who are passionate and personable—and let's face it,
they are trying to weed out the arrogant, the socially
dysfunctional, the total jerks. I heard about one appli-
cant this year who found himself in a group interview
situation—four applicants, all presumably sitting there
thinking, *they're only going to take one of us, they're only going to take one of us!* And sure enough, one of the four decided to play the jerk: he mentioned his own Ivy League
pedigree a mere eight or nine times, he looked visibly
bored and disgusted when the other students spoke, he
insulted their answers. Imagine how easy he made it for
the interviewers; we all know what kind of medical student that guy will make. He was saying, loud and clear,

take me and I will be one of the class jerks! I could name
you his equivalents in my own class so long ago, and I
could tell you their medical school nicknames too, except that they're unprintable. We all know from our experience of doctors that the weeding-out process is
imperfect, but there it is: They are picking some hundred young people in whom to invest their energy, their
time, their cadavers, and their imprimatur. They don't
want to waste spaces on creeps. If they take you, they in-
tend to make a doctor of you.

Medical training is transformative. It will make you
over completely—your emotions, your sense of propor-
tion, your narrative abilities, and your habits of mind.
The process starts in college, as you make the choice to
be premed and spend your college years under a certain
amount of pressure. But it's when you get to medical
school that the real transformation begins. I will try to
pin down some of the elements of that transformation as
we go forward, try to help you see why medical training
is more than just assimilating a great deal of information.
It also involves assimilating responsibility, and making
what we can only call life-and-death part of your daily
routine. Maybe this sense of suddenly mixing with life
and death is part of why we often compare medical
training to military training, why you hear the expres-
sions, "basic training," or "in the trenches." It means accepting pain and disease as your familiars, and remaking

many of your normal and proper responses to life (yes, I want to see what's under that bandage—yes, I want to be in that room where the people pulled from that terrible car crash have been brought—yes, I want to be there when we tell the patient he has cancer). And it means changing your sense of identification; I promise you that when you come out of this training, you will in some sense divide the world into doctors and non-doctors, and you will identify as a doctor.

One convention of medical education is that many classes and discussion sessions and conferences begin with a medical case: *Twenty-eight-year-old male of Mediterranean heritage presents with pallor and lethargy. The patient states that he was well until four days ago, when he began feeling tired and was unable to go about his usual activities. He denies any fever, arthralgias, or myalgias. . . .*

The really good test takers among you should have made the correct diagnosis in the first sentence: *Why are they bothering to tell us that he's of Mediterranean heritage? Must have some significance. Which diseases are disproportionately present in that group? Got it—he has G6PD deficiency and something has made him hemolyze!* In other words, you think the patient in the vignette has an inherited enzyme deficiency—he doesn't have enough glucose-6-phosphate dehydrogenase. And in the presence of certain medications or certain foods (most famously fava beans), people with this enzyme deficiency start to hemolyze, to chew up their own red blood cells, and as they destroy their red blood cells, they can become severely anemic. So then you read on to see if there are any other clues. . . . *The patient states that five days ago he was having back pain, and took some unknown medication provided by his brother-in-law* . . . Bingo! There we are. He has G6PD deficiency and he took some medication that set him off and now he's hemolyzing!

Medical education keeps building on these cases. Sometimes they will ask you what would be your first action. Sometimes they take you through the whole course of the illness, step by step. When I have to recertify in pediatrics, every seven years, I take a long multiple-choice test, and there are those same case descriptions. So you might as well get used to them. After a while, it becomes second nature to formulate the people you meet, the patients you see, in that way. You're beginning to learn to tell a medical story. As you progress through medical school, you will learn a whole new vocabulary, even a jargon, and a new set of nicknames and abbreviations. You'll even learn some new grammar and sentence structure. At first it will sound strange to hear yourself speaking in this way: *"This forty-five-year-old female, gravida 4, para 3, SAB 1, status/post outpatient surgery four days prior to admission for menorrhagia, now presents with chest pain, rule-out MI. . . ."* (She's forty-five, she's been pregnant four times, had three children and one miscarriage [SAB, spontaneous abortion], four days ago she had surgery for heavy menstrual bleeding, and now she's here with chest pain and we're worried she might be having a heart attack [MI, myocardial infarction]). I promise you that by the time you graduate, you also will be past master at constructing these formalized stories, these information-packed clinical vignettes. Of course, as you get to know your patients well, you will become increasingly aware of what these formalized narratives leave out, even as you become efficient at assembling them.

All your training in medicine is supposed to lead to this, to the ability to interpret the clues and put the pieces together and figure out a particular patient. I started this letter by considering you as the patient—anxious, drinking too much coffee, obsessing over your e-mail, having trouble sleeping, dreaming of white coats and stethoscopes. And as we consider your case, we imagine hands popping up around the room as eager-beaver medical students comment on the symptoms, the diagnosis, and the management. Avid to use medical jargon, one student comments that this illness is iatrogenic, a word that means an illness caused by the medical profession. Iatrogenic infections, for example, are the ones that patients acquire in the hospital, or as a consequence of medical procedures. Yes, chimes in a classmate, also eager to use medical terms, it's iatrogenic and it can have a high morbidity, but a low mortality. By that she means your condition can cause you all kinds of harm but is unlikely to kill you. But at least, she goes on, it's usually self-limiting, and in most cases, it resolves spontaneously. The medical students nod, thinking a little of their own trajectories. They, after all, have all experienced some variant of the stresses now afflicting you, and they do remember those days. On the other hand, now that they are in medical school, life has not exactly relaxed. Yes, they know they're going to be doctors, they know they've made it in—though many of them probably have moments every now and then of expecting to be kicked out, to be told it's all been a mistake, bad idea, go on home and find something else to do with your life. On top of that anxiety, and the pressures of huge amounts of material to learn and tests to take, and the constant smell of formaldehyde permeating their clothing, many of them are probably prey to the classic medical student anxiety in which you keep diagnosing yourself with all the terrible diseases you study, you keep identifying your own risk factors and your symptoms. That's what the student is thinking of who considers your case and offers up the comment that indeed your condition is generally self-resolving, but it is well known that it can sometimes be a precursor to another iatrogenic self-limited condition, medical student syndrome. But the pressures and the information overload that bring on these conditions also offer you relief: The more you learn, and the more you apply that knowledge to patients, real or theoretical, the less absorbed you are likely to be in your own woes and symptoms. Maturity, for a medical student, involves understanding that your own case—however interesting it may be to you—is not what the story is really about.

## 2

■ Asking Questions,
Crossing Borders

*This forty-six-year-old white male was admitted with an extensive skin infection on his left leg; on admission, he was noted to be speaking loudly, and described seeing things that were not there; on exam, he was tremulous, with tachycardia and generally unstable vital signs, and a tongue lag. He states that he is currently homeless, living in a shelter, and that his health is generally excellent. In the emergency room, he admitted to smoking half a pack per day and occasionally drinking "two or three beers." He is currently complaining of severe leg pain, which he attributes to the skin infection, and he is requesting medications for pain control. He will require significant care on discharge from the hospital, but states that he has no family members who can care for him.*

*Dear Orlando,*

Would you know how to talk to a patient like this? Would you know how to ask him about the life he's led? Would you know how to understand his answers? Would you see past his statement that he drinks the occasional beer or two, and realize—from the way he is acting, from his unstable vital signs, from his physical exam— that he is in danger of going into acute alcohol withdrawal, a potentially life-threatening condition? When you read that clinical vignette, do you find yourself angry at the guy, blaming him for his situation in life? If you realized he is an alcoholic, do you see his drinking as somewhere on a continuum with drinking you know of, say among college students—the kind of drinking I am always warning you about? Do you think it's related to your parents enjoying their martinis? Or does it fall in some completely different category? He's your patient, this homeless alcoholic gentleman—do you feel some strong sense of kinship, or some troubling sense of distance? I assume that you believe medical school can teach you how to diagnose and treat his skin infection— and presumably also how to recognize and treat his alcohol withdrawal. But have you ever stopped to wonder how on earth medical school can teach you to listen to his story and understand anything of his life?

Last September, as part of my faculty responsibilities at NYU Medical School, I went to the first meeting of a course for all the first-year medical students. I looked around the room, and what I thought first was, *my god, they're so young*. And then, *my god, I'm so old*. But they aren't really so young. They're mostly new college graduates or people who've been out of college a few years—young men and women in their twenties. People this age step into all kinds of jobs: They staff legislators' offices in Washington; they fill the lower-echelon jobs in publishing and finance; and heaven knows they fill the military—they carry weapons, they fight and die. But that room of first-month-of-their-first-year medical students had a special quality of youth. They looked *impressed*. They were dressed like college students, all right, in jeans and sandals and T-shirts and sweatshirts that revealed their undergraduate or hometown or baseball loyalties. Only the occasional light blue scrub shirt, probably on a student outfitted for gross anatomy, set any medical tone at all. They lounged in the auditorium seats and kicked their backpacks out of the way so they could stretch out their legs, and they joked and flirted with one another. But they looked very, well, impressed. Something about the first year of medical school had already rocked them, unsettled them.

The first year of medical school is supposed to do that. That's one reason many schools start you right off with gross anatomy, the course that, among all others, is designed to let you know that you're in the army now, so to speak. If cutting into a cadaver doesn't tell you that you are finally and truly a medical student, then whatever could? There's definitely a certain sense, in that first year of medical school, that they're breaking you down a little bit, in order to reconstruct you in the image of a doctor. You know, Orlando, I feel a little strange saying this to you—and saying it in a way that makes it sound like I approve. "Breaking you down a little bit." I don't want you broken down. I want your training to add to you and build on the skills and the interests you already have. And yet I know that some part of what medical school will do to you will go beyond that, that it will unmake you as well as make you, and that part of that process of unmaking you is that new sense you acquire, by actually taking apart a body, of how we are all made.

But this wasn't gross anatomy. There were no dead bodies covered with sheets, waiting to be dissected. For that matter, there was no backbreaking load of arcane information to be memorized and assimilated, no make-or-break two-hundred-question exam in the offing in this particular course. It was a course on the relationship between the physician and the patient, and the first part would focus on talking to patients. Four of these first-year students would be my tutorial group; we would meet every couple of weeks and together the five of us would sit down with a patient—a hospitalized patient, a clinic patient, any willing patient I could find. The students would ask questions, and then it would be my job to go over the whole interaction with them—what had they asked, what had they learned, what had they understood.

It wasn't my job—or the job of this course—to teach the formal art of the patient interview, the codified lists of questions that you will need to learn in order to "take a medical history." You can't teach those questions to students who don't know any anatomy or pathophysiology; what would be the point of memorizing a long list of questions about the exact location and nature of chest pain, back pain, neck pain, if you don't yet know anything about angina or aortic aneurysms or gastroesophageal reflux? No, my job was just to help my tutorial group learn to ask questions and begin to think about how you understand a patient's story. They weren't responsible for taking a formal medical history, and heaven knows they weren't supposed to formulate a treatment plan. So why did they look so nervous?

Courses like this one represent a major change in medical education. We are trying now, in medical school, to bring patients in earlier, to leaven the basic science with clinical reality. It used to be that the individual you got to know best in your first year was your cadaver, and that you received specific instruction on teasing out the nerves of a dead body, but you heard nothing about teasing out the details of a living person's life. That was supposed to wait for the clinical years—the third and fourth years in which, stuffed full of physiology and pathophysiology, you would finally be allowed onto "the wards" to deal with patients. Medical students have been complaining for a long time that they wanted more clinical contacts in their first years of school. And patients have been complaining even longer that many doctors are not good at talking and asking questions and listening to answers. Medical education doesn't change quickly, but it does change, and it has changed to deal with these two imperatives: to teach students more formally and more carefully about the art of asking and listening and observing, and to build their training more and more around patients—the fictitious patients in the clinical vignettes, and the real patients who can actually answer you back.

A couple of decades ago, when I was a medical student, the only "patient contact" programmed into our first year took place during the clinical sessions that were part of the big lecture courses: A patient, invited for this occasion, would stand at the podium beside the professor and talk about what it was like to live with sickle cell disease or neurofibromatosis or cancer. About what it was like to live through the operation that the professor had just described, or to take the medications we had just carefully copied down into our notes. One hundred and fifty students, one professor, one patient. These patients were hand-picked and invited by our professors specifically because they had so much to teach us. Many of them were highly articulate—they had chosen to speak to us because they thought it was important for us to understand what they and their families had been through.

Some of them were angry at the medical system and wanted us to know it.

As medical students we were desperate for patient contact. After college and the intense premed years, after all the multiple-choice exams and applications and essays and interviews, here we finally were, on track to do what most of us had been dreaming about since childhood. This was medicine, this was the stuff that would make us doctors. Every patient was a reminder that this information was more than science, more than another academic hurdle. This information would allow us to touch people, to touch their lives.

But for most of that first year of medical school, we felt removed from patient care and even from medicine itself. We were, above all, professional students, as you are now, after four years of being a college premed. Like you, we had made it through the premed courses by perfecting the ability to study, to memorize, to cram, to take one exam and then hit the ground running toward the next. And the first year of medical school felt like a frantic test of all those skills. Okay, so you think you are a good memorizer: Now learn all the muscles of the arms and shoulders and torso, now learn the blood vessels, now memorize the nerves!

Back then, the first year was about studying and study guides and study questions, textbooks and handouts, staying up too late and devising magic sentences and mnemonics to help you remember the bones of the foot, or the twelve cranial nerves, or maybe the Krebs cycle, that series of equations essential for understanding energy use in living cells. (Medical students are famous for their off-color mnemonics. For example, there are 12 cranial nerves, which need to be remembered in their proper order; you can learn their names with a magic sentence too obscene to be printed here. But then you have to learn whether nerves I–XII are sensory, motor, or both, and one mnemonic for that is "Some Say Marry Money, But My Brother Says Big Breasts Matter More.")

When you enter medical school, you are eager to learn about disease and how to cure it. But before you can understand what happens when the body comes apart or stops functioning, you have to understand how it's put together and how it functions in proper detail, so you spend much of the first year of medical school studying "the normal." Anatomy and pathophysiology and biochemistry and histology—these are the chemical equations that power the cell in biochemistry, these are the three kinds of muscle cells, up close and personal under a microscope in histology, here is physiology with the details of how nerves transmit signals and how muscles contract. Then in gross anatomy, there are all the muscles and their relations and insertions and their blood vessels and nerves to be dissected out and memorized. In the second year, you tackle pathophysiology, and you learn what happens when things go wrong. I'm not sure that I could see it when I was a medical student, but when I think about it now, the plan had a certain grand and glorious sweep: first come to know the body inside out, appreciate this remarkable machine in which you live, and then begin, system by system, to consider what happens when it breaks down. If you really grasp this knowledge, it will change your view of yourself and of everyone else. It is another way of changing you, of taking you apart a little, as you take apart your cadaver, and then reassembling you.

But I didn't experience those first two years of medical school as a rich and layered approach to essential knowledge. Most of the time, it felt like huge slices of knowledge assembled and handed over to be learned, not always in any obvious order, and sometimes just to be learned on faith that some day this would all be useful. I understand now that much of this was my own fault—that I didn't appreciate how useful this information would be to me someday because I hadn't yet made the imaginative leap of really seeing myself as a doctor, as someone whose knowledge of the body—and of this body of knowledge—would be directly useful and helpful every day. So I'm not particularly proud of all the whining I did—about the rote learning and the poorly organized courses and the lack of clinical relevance.

As it happens, though, in 1986, just as my class was graduating from Harvard Medical School, the school unveiled with great fanfare a new curriculum. Finally, medical school was going to stop relying on large and unconnected lecture courses and would instead teach students in smaller groups and center the learning on patients and problems. This completely revamped million-dollar curriculum was called the New Pathway. And our deans happily gave interviews to the newspapers about everything that was wrong with the medical education for which my classmates and I had just gone deeply into debt.

The spirit that guided those curriculum reforms has meant changes in many medical schools. And when you study medicine today, like those first-year NYU medical students I met in the fall of 2006, you are likely to encounter a more coordinated curriculum, a more thought-out approach—and a great deal more effort devoted to clinical relevance and patient contact in the first two years. The basic structure remains the same: a year spent learning normal processes, a year spent learning pathophysiology, and then two years out "on the wards," moving from internal medicine to surgery to pediatrics to OB to neurology to any subspecialty that interests you, watching doctors as they practice and you yourself—yes, you—talking to patients and touching patients and finally getting to wear that white coat.

But there's a problem. As I have pointed out, first-year medical students don't necessarily know anything—in September a first-year medical student knows exactly as much as a premed college senior in June, or maybe a little less, allowing for the natural processes of entropy and forgetfulness. So you can't give them any responsibility for patient care. There are some first-year medical students who know a lot—one guy in my tutorial group trained as an EMT, and you would be lucky if he were standing nearby when you happened to have a heart attack. And there are first-year students who have already had careers as nurses, or who have spent time delivering babies and helping with emergency surgery in third-world hospitals. But most first-year medical students are pretty green.

In my first year in medical school, I remember a fourth-year student telling us what to do if we were ever on an airplane and someone started having chest pain. You'll be sitting there, said the lecturer, and you'll think you should offer to help—after all, you're a medical student—and you'll feel terrible because you won't know what to do. So I'm going to tell you what to do, she said. First, wait for a half minute and see if a doctor speaks up—a *real* doctor. If not, go reassure the passenger, and ask a few questions. Has he had heart trouble? Does he take nitroglycerin? If he does, have him take one. If he says he doesn't have one with him, have the flight attendants ask if anyone else on the plane can give him one. Then ask them to get him extra oxygen. Then tell the pilot to land the plane as soon as possible. You'll have done what you can do. And I remember writing it all down, every word. I was desperate for competence and assurance and a sense that I could actually come through in a crisis. To tell you the truth, I still worry about something like this coming up on an airplane; my pediatric skills are unlikely to come in very handy, but I worry that there will be an adult having a heart attack—not something with which I have a great deal of experience. I was once on an airplane, waiting to take off, when a man across the aisle began to have chest pain—and dutifully, I told the flight attendant that I was a physician—and I began to rehearse in my mind the instructions of that long-ago first-year lecture, crossed with the specifics for adult CPR, just in case. Fortunately, the flight attendant told me not to worry; we were simply going to return to the gate and the EMTs were waiting.

I thought about this the first time I met with my tutorial group, my four first-year students. I thought about how desperate I had once been for a few tricks and shortcuts that I hoped would convince all bystanders that I was a real doctor, ready to save lives and take care of patients. My job with my tutorial group had a different goal: to encourage them to acknowledge the newness and strangeness of their role, and to help them take those first steps in interviewing patients, rather than preparing to rush right past all the preliminaries to heroic action. I was to escort them to their first patient interviews and help them ask questions and understand the answers. We wouldn't spend our time on the kind of patient-by-patient, problem-by-problem learning that is what the third and fourth years are all about. Instead, they would try to understand how to talk to strangers about their lives and their medical problems—and how to put together and understand the stories. I would try to draw valuable lessons for them from those first patient interviews.

The first lesson I learned, all over again, is how big a deal this is. When you walk into a room and begin asking questions, when you start "interviewing" a patient, you are stepping across a border. Medical training is full of borders you need to cross. Gross anatomy is a major dividing line; right there, in your first year, you do something that most people never do, something that every doctor has done: you painstakingly dissect a dead body, and you learn to name and trace and locate all its parts (how long you remember this information is another interesting question, and we'll get to that later on). Learning how to do a physical exam is a big-time border crossing—there you are, touching other people's bodies in a new and professional way, grappling with the taboos of modesty and sexuality, as well as the whole grand history of the laying on of hands and what that means.

We'll talk about that later, too.

There are many other physical boundaries you learn to breach—from drawing blood to making a surgical incision to inserting a medical instrument. But what my tutorial group was teaching me last fall was that just asking questions is by itself full of power and magic and tension and strangeness. I had forgotten that. Over the past twenty years, I've walked into so many rooms to start versions of this medical conversation—with patients I know well, with total strangers, with people in pain, with people unwilling to tell me what's really wrong, with people who can't stop telling me what's wrong—I've come to take it for granted.

It was clear that none of the people in my tutorial group took this for granted in any way. This was a big deal: an interview with a real patient. They had listened carefully to the course guidelines; they were dressed professionally (no T-shirts, no sandals), they were not carrying big bags or backpacks, which might take up too much space in a patient's small room, and they were wearing their short white jackets. In medicine, a short white coat denotes a person in training, as opposed to the knee-length white coat of the full-fledged physician. But all white coats are heavy with symbolism—in recent years, many medical schools have begun having a white coat ceremony at the beginning of the first year, a ritual in which these short white coats are issued as a mark of professionalism—another border crossing.

My students were wearing their white coats to show they were on their way to being doctors. I, on the other hand, was not wearing a white coat, although I have several of those nice long ones in my closet. Pediatricians, and especially primary-care pediatricians, tend not to wear them, because many small children, who have had a few go-rounds with immunization, will simply start screaming at the sight of a white coat. Then you can just say goodbye to any chance of observing the child's development or listening to the heart or the lungs.

The person the medical students were going to interview was the grandmother of a ten-year-old girl who was in the pediatric intensive care unit, or PICU. In pediatrics, a patient interview often means a parent interview. You always talk to the child if the child can talk, but this child couldn't talk; she had been in a catastrophic car accident and remained in a coma. I wanted the students to get a sense of the life her grandmother was living. The grandmother was the child's guardian, she was from out of town, and she was essentially living in the hospital, sleeping in the family room, bathing in the hospital bathroom. I wanted the students to get a sense of what an injury like this can do to an entire family. I wanted them to get a sense of how the grandmother understood the prognosis, and a sense of the interactions she had had with the doctors and the nurses during this long hospitalization. The head of the unit had recommended her, saying she was pleasant and articulate and had a lot of time on her hands, since she was essentially living in the PICU. And so the day before, I had asked her if she would be willing to talk with us.

Ever since my residency, I have been fascinated by the parents, usually mothers, who find themselves living these shadow lives in the hospital when a child is sick for

a long time. As a resident, I sometimes felt that *I* lived in
the hospital. Wasn't I there at all hours? Wasn't I an expert at all the peculiar hallway connections and service
elevators? Didn't I know the cafeteria schedule by heart,
and couldn't I locate emergency sources of food when
the cafeteria was closed, from vending machines to the
ward kitchens where there were stashes of saltines
wrapped in cellophane and cardboard cups of ice cream,
intended for the patients? Wasn't I all too familiar with
the feel of the call-room mattress and pillow; didn't I
know how, in my sleep, to adjust the fixtures on a hospital shower and blast myself awake with hot water? It was
something of an affectation, something of a boast, and
something of a complaint: I am truly a resident, in every
sense; I live here, I belong here. And then as I moved
through the hospital—my hospital—I would become
aware of these resident mothers, living in their ailing
children's rooms, keeping their vigils, and I would feel
put in my place, self-dramatizing and foolish.

In fact, Orlando, as you know, there were a couple of
weeks when I actually *was* a parent who lived in the hospital as well as a resident: that awful summer when you
fractured your femur, and you spent two weeks in trac-
tion in a hospital bed in my hospital. And I just stopped
going home; I worked all day and sometimes all night as
a resident, and then, when things were quiet, I went to
your room and tried to sleep on the chair provided for
parents, which unfolded into a bed. I did it for two

weeks, and then I took home an essentially intact child, even if you were in a body cast. And I wondered more than ever about the resident parents on the oncology ward, or the neurosurgery ward. How did they keep body and soul together, how did they manage in the hospital week after week after week?

When I asked the grandmother whether she would be willing to talk to my tutorial group, I told her in particular that I wanted them to understand her experience of living in the hospital, and she nodded. I figured that this approach would provide us with material that would be educational for the students but not too highly fraught or emotional for the grandmother.

The four students and the grandmother and I took our places around a small table. I planned to start off by making introductions, by telling her the names of the students. I would thank her for speaking to us, I would model good manners for the medical students by addressing her formally—calling her Mrs. So-and-so—and I would model honesty for the students by making it perfectly clear that they were students, not doctors. And then, since it was their first interview, I would gently steer things in the direction of that living-in-the-hospital question. But as it happened, I had no chance to say a word, or to model anything at all, let alone to steer, gently or ungently.

Our interview subject must have been thinking about this encounter ever since we had made the appointment

twenty-four hours earlier. She began to speak even before we had taken our seats. A small, solid woman, she
leaned forward and stared intently at the medical students, one by one. "I am the grandmother of the ten-
year-old girl who was hit by a truck," she began, and
gave them the date of the accident, and some of the
other medical details. From then on, she held the floor. I
did not introduce the students, and for the first fifteen
minutes of the interview, they did not have any chance to
ask their questions. The grandmother talked. Sentences
poured out—the terrible day of the accident, the hours
in the emergency room, the head trauma, the broken
limbs. The intensive care unit, the surgeries, the set-
backs, the infections, the complications. But in a sense,
she hurried through the story of the child's current medical condition, though she clearly knew everything there
was to know. She wanted us to know what her granddaughter had been through, to shake our heads over the
extent of her injuries, to admire the strength with which
the child had held on tight to life, and was now even beginning to make some progress toward recovery. But this
grandmother had a different story that mattered even
more to her, and she wanted to tell it and retell it. We
needed to know about her granddaughter as she had
been before the accident—about the life the two of them
had led together, about their daily routine, and her
granddaughter's happy and affectionate personality. She

wanted to tell us what her granddaughter used to say every morning, about how joyful each new day made her feel, about the hugs and kisses, about how the child had danced through life—before the accident.

We sat there, the four first-year medical students and me. None of us wanted to interrupt her or redirect her, and I'm not sure it would have been possible. I was uncomfortably conscious that they were supposed to practice asking questions, and I was also aware that, without meaning to, I had thrown them into a situation so fraught with intense emotion and tragic overtones that it might be too much for a first patient encounter. But I was also thinking to myself that at least this would teach them the most important lesson of clinical medicine: *All of this is real. All of this is serious. These are real people with real feelings, and being a doctor inserts you into their lives at the moments of highest drama and sharpest anxiety and deepest sorrow—and that comes with the territory.* We were sitting in a room with someone's terrible, terrible tragedy—and trying to learn from it. I'm sure the students felt a little bit, well, parasitic, because I know I did. Was it really right to ask this woman to go down into the valley of her sorrows for our sake, was it fair to put her through this, did we have any right to be here at all? Yet I remembered how willingly she had agreed to meet with us; I thought about how she had apparently been planning what to say. And I told myself that at least the medical students could learn one essential lesson here: When you can't do anything else, listen and pay attention.

The medical students did very well. They sat and they listened, and they obviously felt for this woman and her beloved devastated child. After a while, they began to ask questions: What has it been like for you, living here while your granddaughter is in the hospital? What was it like that first day in the emergency room, right after the accident? One of them asked a really good question: Where have you found the strength to carry on like this? And the grandmother told them about the hospital chapel, where she went every day to pray. They asked about the rest of her life, and she told them pieces of her story, a hard story, full of taking care of other people— her mother, her children, her grandchildren.

But no matter what questions the students asked, the grandmother kept veering back to her memories of the happy, laughing, blessed child she had known before the accident. She wanted us to meet that child—that child no one might recognize again, that child who might never again recognize anyone. She wanted us to see and hear and understand that little girl, to recognize her and remember her. And finally, after we had been sitting and talking for forty minutes, as she was telling us again about the smile of delight with which her granddaughter had greeted each new morning, about how much she had loved school and what a good student she had been, finally, the grandmother broke down and began to sob, still looking straight at the medical students.

We sat frozen for a second or two, and then I jumped up to get tissues. Thank you for telling us about your granddaughter, we said, thank you so much for helping us understand, thank you for being so generous with us. And she took a tissue and she stopped crying, and we talked a little longer, and then we all thanked her and we walked with her over to the PICU, to stand with her at the bedside of the little girl, her fractured limbs in casts, her chest rising and falling with the ventilator breaths. And then we said goodbye, and the four medical students and I went back to sit together and discuss this, our first clinical interview.

I explained about some of the medical supports we had seen in the PICU and talked a little about how hard it is to give a prognosis in a situation like this. But the students wanted a prognosis, or they wanted me to tell them there was a good chance the little girl would recover. And I wanted to tell them that because I wanted it to be true. Children have amazing powers of resilience, I said, which is part of the glory of pediatrics. That was true. Children can come back from terrible disasters, I said, but it's hard to predict, and this child has a long, hard road in front of her. We talked about the grandmother's spirit, about the importance of her faith, about the logistics of her hospital life, sleeping in the family room, bathing in the patient bathroom, praying in the hospital chapel.

We talked about the interview itself, which had been so loaded with emotion, and so difficult. No matter how good a student you are, and how much biology and chemistry and gross anatomy you have learned, this is a real border you cross. When you sit in a room with a real person and ask that person questions, you cross into a new zone, a zone in which you are being permitted, even required, to do something most people will never do. Even in a high-tech age of miraculous imaging that takes you inside the body, there is something overwhelmingly powerful about that patient interview, about finding yourself face-to-face with that other person and preparing yourself to understand that person's story. It is the oldest and most basic doctor-patient encounter, the piece that happens even before the laying on of hands, and it retains its impact. It rocks you and it shakes you and it brings you up against all your own limitations, all your self-consciousness, all your uncertainty.

As the semester went on, my group and I met with a whole range of patients, including that guy in the vignette that opens this chapter. We talked about how you might ask someone for more detail about his drinking, even if he didn't happen to think that his drinking had much to do with why he was in the hospital. About how you might try to find out exactly how a patient with severe diabetes understood her disease, how you might get her to describe the symptoms that let her know her blood sugar was a little high or a little low. We asked a man with severe cerebral palsy whether there was something in particular he wanted the medical students to hear. He answered that he wanted them to know that people with disabilities—people like him—could fall in love just like anyone else. And we heard other patients echo what the grandmother had told us about the importance of religion in their lives.

The students in my tutorial were overwhelmed by the experience of interviewing that grandmother. Her eloquence, her intensity, and then finally her weeping had done them in. They wanted to do something to comfort her, just as they wanted me to promise them that her granddaughter would get better.

"So is it okay to hug a patient?" one of the students asked. I thought about it. He was maybe twenty-two years old, deeply moved, respectful, and eager to comfort. After all, I had put my arm around the grandmother when I offered the tissues. Was that okay? Was it okay for him to hug? The most honest answer I could give was that it was *probably* okay for *me* to hug this particular woman. "I'm only a few years younger than she is," I said, thinking aloud. "I have a kid around her granddaughter's age—I'm a woman—I thought she wanted some kind of physical comfort, not a real hug, but a hand on her shoulder. I don't think there was any way she could have misinterpreted it. I'm not sure it would be okay for a twenty-two-year-old guy to hug her. But you do have to find ways of comforting people and acknowledging their grief."

"Does it get easier?" another student asked me. "Do you get used to things like this?"

At first I wanted to say no, of course not, how could you get used to things like this? But the truth is more complicated. I have sat with so many grief-stricken or terror-stricken parents and grandparents. I have reassured and I have comforted, but I have also broken bad news—sometimes the worst news that someone will ever hear.

*When we did the spinal tap, we found meningitis.*

*Your baby has HIV.*

*We did our best, but your son didn't make it.*

In some profound way, I have come to think of this as part of my job—not a happy part, and certainly not a part I look forward to, but also not a part that I would wish away. Going into medicine is deciding to line yourself up on the side of the real and the serious, choosing to be in a profession that will insert you, again and again, into these moments when people's lives change, or unravel, or come together, or turn suddenly and sharply in a new and often unwelcome direction. I have learned to protect myself a little—to understand that the tragedy is happening to the patient, and not to me, and that my job is to focus on the patient and on helping, not on my own emotions. I believe the woman we had just interviewed understood that she was talking to four people who were setting off along this path.

I stayed in touch with the grandmother over the next week or so, and indeed there were small hopeful bits of progress to celebrate. In fact, because the child was significantly more stable from a medical point of view, she was transferred to a rehabilitation hospital much closer to home, where her long and difficult story will continue. This grandmother had been so gracious and generous with herself, speaking to the students at a moment of terrible stress and uncertainty and sorrow. And I believe she spoke to them as she did because she wanted them to take with them—in the ever-expanding file of clinical memories that all doctors carry—a picture of her granddaughter, as she once had been, dancing into the kitchen to give her grandmother a good-morning kiss.

# 3

## ▓ Physical Findings: Appreciating a Mass

*A full-term 3.2 kg male infant born yesterday by spontaneous vaginal delivery was discovered on physical examination to have a right-sided abdominal mass. The baby is otherwise well-appearing, pink and vigorous, with no rashes, normal facies without anomalies, no lymphadenopathy, normal cardiac exam, S1 and S2 without murmurs or gallops, abdomen soft and nontender with the mass palpable in the right upper quadrant. . . .*

*Dear Orlando,*

I remember once when I was a resident, working in the newborn nursery, one of the neonatology fellows came in and excitedly announced that he had felt a mass in a baby's abdomen. This was a guy who had already chosen to devote his life to newborns—he had finished his three-year residency in pediatrics, and now he was doing a three-year fellowship in neonatology. His days and nights were spent covering high-risk deliveries, working in the newborn intensive care unit, doing research in newborn medicine. In other words, he had already examined many newborns. But this was the first time he had felt an abdominal mass that he had not expected to feel.

Let me tell you about feeling a mass—in a baby's belly or in a woman's breast or even in a man's testicle. It's not exactly the distinct certain aha-there-it-is moment that you probably imagine. Over and over, in your medical training, people will teach you how to examine the squishier parts of the body, checking for masses. Whole books have been written on the palpation of the abdomen—that is, feeling the belly. There's an art and a science to examining a newborn's belly even after you know the drill through and through. First you observe— you look at the abdomen to see if there are any irregularities or discolorations—and frankly, with babies at least, there is almost never anything to see. Then you listen with your stethoscope to hear bowel sounds, because once you start to press on the abdomen, the baby will begin screaming, and that's the end of your chance to hear anything from inside the intestines. Finally you press— and you press hard. In a newborn baby, you're supposed to press down so deep that you can feel the kidneys, which as you may remember are located all the way back near your spine. I have always had trouble feeling the kidneys, but I tell myself that if there was something abnormal there—like a mass—well, *that* I would surely feel. And so you palpate, pressing firmly down with your fingers, quadrant by quadrant. In the right upper quadrant is the liver, in the left upper quadrant is the spleen, in the lower quadrants are lots of intestines. The entire point of the exercise is to satisfy yourself that there is no mass. And basically, there never is. You can spend hours in the newborn nursery examining newborn after newborn, and odds are you will not find a mass.

But just think about what you are doing, there in the newborn nursery: You are looking at baby after baby after baby, and *you are the first to examine each one.* That's why I'm starting this letter with the idea of examining a newborn—it's not just that I'm a pediatrician, it's that when you look at a brand-new baby, there is always the chance that there is some absolutely vital piece of information there for you. No one has already checked out, certified, written up, and referred this baby. You are embarked on a voyage of discovery, with the small but real possibility that you are going to describe and name an important and unexpected feature of this unexplored landscape.

That was why the neonatology fellow was so excited. He had felt masses before, but they were masses other doctors had discovered. He had never, until that moment, pressed down routinely on a routine baby's stomach and felt something wrong loom up against his fingers. He had made an important discovery: He had used his routine skills, his everyday exam, and it had brought him somewhere new. He felt, I would guess, like a doctor—but in some new and powerful way.

I know what you're probably thinking: This was not good news for the baby. A mass might mean a badly malformed kidney or else a tumor, a neuroblastoma, for example, a rare cancer that can be already in place when a baby is born. A mass in the belly of a perfectly normal-appearing baby changes the whole story, the whole destiny of the child and the family. You might make other life-changing discoveries. You could hear an unusual murmur and end up finding that the baby has a cardiac malformation—more common than the tumors. You could note small, subtle abnormalities—low-set ears, say, or tiny pinpoint sinus openings in front of the ears, or a deep dimple at the base of the spine with a little tuft of hair growing over it, any of which might send you looking for more serious hidden anomalies. Those low-set ears may signal any one of a host of genetic syndromes; that spinal dimple and tuft of hair may signal that the baby has a hidden spina bifida, an opening in the spinal column. When we teach the newborn exam to medical students, we say over and over, undress the baby completely, look at every inch of the skin. Babies aren't that big, I find myself saying, less than brilliantly. You can look at the whole baby.

That's what they teach you about examining adults, too. In medical school I heard a story about a student who examined a patient in a cursory way—pulled the sheet down a little, listened to the guy's heart through his hospital johnny, looked in his eyes and down his throat—and then reported that the physical exam was completely normal. His attending—his supervising doctor—asked him if he had palpated the pedal pulses bilaterally—that is, if he had felt the pulses in both feet to check for circulation. Oh, yes, said the student, showing off, dorsalis pedis and posterior tibialis were normal bilaterally—that is, the pulse at the back of the ankle and the pulse on the top of the foot were normal on the left and on the right. The attending took him to the bedside, folded down the blanket all the way, and revealed that the patient in fact had no right foot—and no right leg either; he had had an above-the-knee amputation years before.

I don't know if this medical student is real or apocryphal—he offers such a valid teaching point that you have to be a little suspicious. But I certainly know how easy it is to cut corners on a physical exam. Sometimes it's for your own convenience: Are you really going to wait while someone takes off all those clothes? Are you going to peel off that bandage to look under it? Sometimes it's for the patient's convenience. Are you going to insist on doing a rectal exam, even if the patient doesn't want one? It may surprise you to know that I don't think this kind of corner-cutting is necessarily bad. I'm not one of your die-hard physical-diagnosis types; there are doctors who have taken good care of me who haven't focused on doing a thorough exam because it wasn't all that relevant to the particular question that brought me in. If I go in with a bad cough and need to know if I have pneumonia, I don't really want to be told to take off my pants. Listen to my lungs carefully, look in my throat, check my lymph nodes, then tell me what you think. Save the rest for my checkup.

But when you don't know a patient, or you don't know what is going on—Why is she so tired all the time? Why is he having those dizzy spells?—then you really do need to go over the person carefully, top to bottom, looking for physical evidence. In pediatrics, there's a classic diagnostic dilemma: the baby or young toddler brought to the emergency room because he won't stop screaming. There's a whole list of possible causes—the classic, before the days of disposable diapers, was an open diaper pin sticking the baby. Screaming and crying are the only way young children have to indicate that something's wrong. The screaming could mean the baby has the kind of belly pain that indicates appendicitis *or* the kind of belly pain that means gas. It could also mean an eyelash is in the eye, or a hair from the head has fallen out and become wound tightly around a toe, cutting off circulation. Or maybe the baby has an ear infection, and he's crying because there's pressure building up behind his eardrum, or maybe it's just a sore hangnail. You go over and over babies like that, looking for some explanation of their distress—and sometimes you find something, and sometimes you just worry, and sometimes the baby magically quiets down while he's waiting to have his stomach x-rayed. You're x-raying his stomach because after you've given up on everything else, you think maybe that when you pressed all the way down on his belly, maybe, just maybe, you felt something.

Examining other people's bodies is another one of those borders you learn to cross in your medical training. You take a class in physical diagnosis, or in introduction to clinical medicine, and you start out by examining other medical students, listening to a classmate's lungs with your brand-new stethoscope, or standing behind someone, delicately positioning your fingers around the front of her throat and attempting to palpate her thyroid. I happen to have a thick neck, and I was palpated by any number of my classmates. I don't say they were actually hoping to find a goiter, but I'm sure they would have been thrilled, in the nicest possible way, to come upon what we call a physical finding, an abnormality, a problem detected by physical examination skills. After a few such exams, I was nervous enough to get someone to draw blood and check my thyroid hormone levels. Once I knew they were normal, I could relax and let my classmates palpate. Orlando, when you're learning the physical exam, if you come home on vacation and you'd like to check my thyroid, feel free.

You don't generally ask your classmates to remove any of their clothing. That you do with total strangers—people the age of your parents or your grandparents—or occasionally people your own age. (For the most highly fraught parts of the physical exam, the genital exam, we learned on "models," professional teachers who were paid to let medical students examine them, and who gave us feedback, sometimes stern feedback if we weren't gentle enough or if we examined the wrong place. There's nothing like having the professional patient look you in the eye and say, "Warm that speculum under running water, buddy, before you bring it anywhere near me!" Or maybe, "That's not the ovary, for heaven's sake. You're nowhere near the ovary—stop pressing on my bladder!") This is another of those taboos you have to break over and over until it really feels like it's yours to break, your proper place, your right, to walk into a room, ask a stranger all those intimate questions, and then move on to a careful exam of that stranger's body.

I would like to be pontificating here about the importance of the physical exam. I would like to be telling you the kind of thing I heard over and over during my own training, about the way that a carefully done physical, after a really well-done patient interview, can allow you to make all kinds of important diagnoses and skip all kinds of unnecessary tests and diagnostic procedures. I remember a senior cardiologist taking us through the careful detective work of physical diagnosis—the appearance of the patient's neck veins, the visible appearance of the heart beating beneath the chest, the many different qualities and sounds that could be appreciated through the stethoscope. When you listen to the heart, you can hear so much more than that lub-dub, lub-dub—or at least, he could. The spoken or unspoken message of my teachers was that much of the technology we now have to look at hearts is superfluous, if only you learn to listen carefully. Examine the patient carefully, listen to the patient's heart, think it through, and you'll know what's going on without doing an echocardiogram—a sophisticated ultrasound.

But many doctors—and I'm one of them—can't hear much of what we're supposed to hear. When I listen to someone's heart, I can detect the lub and the dub, I can assess how fast the heart is beating, I can tell if it's beating regularly, and I can hear a nice loud murmur. We score murmurs for loudness from I to VI, and my basic rule of thumb for scoring is always, if I can hear it at all, it's at least a II/VI. If I can hear it clearly, I send the child to a cardiologist, and the cardiologist does an echocardiogram.

So what does all this say about the place of technology in medicine today? In fact, none of us are as good at physical diagnosis as we used to be, because the technology has become more and more available, and by answering our questions quickly and definitely, it has made some of those precious listening and looking and evaluating skills seem less essential, less critical, less a point of professional pride and a matter of life and death.

Don't get me wrong. Almost every field in medicine still cherishes its physical diagnosis skills. Most cardiologists can tell you an enormous amount from listening to your heart—but they still do echocardiograms. Surgeons tend to be unbelievably good at the belly exam—but you probably remember, Orlando, that when your little brother was nine and had mysterious right-sided abdominal pain that woke him up in the middle of the night, he got a lot of belly exams in the emergency room, but he also got a complex CT scan to help the surgeons decide whether or not he had appendicitis. When I was a resident, if you were asked about the utility of radiology in diagnosing appendicitis, the correct answer was to say that it could sometimes be helpful, but it wasn't reliable. Appendicitis was a clinical diagnosis; if the surgeon thought by clinical exam that the patient had it, the surgeon had to take him to the operating room and open him up—only to find, in a certain percentage of cases, that the diagnosis was wrong and the appendix was perfectly healthy. In fact, we were taught that unless surgeons opened up a certain percentage of abdomens to find nothing wrong, they weren't doing enough operations—they were in danger of missing real cases of appendicitis because their index of suspicion was too low. Now radiologists can do an appendiceal CT scan, together with special contrast solutions given "from below" (that is, by enema) and sometimes "from above" (orally), and the study is so reliable that the surgeons feel comfortable relying on it. My son didn't have appendicitis, but I am sure that without all this imaging, they would have taken him to the operating room and opened him up. Instead, the surgeon studied the CT scan and told me he could see evidence of a different problem, omental torsion—a fold of tissue in the abdomen twists on itself, so the blood supply is cut off, causing severe pain. But if you leave it alone, the body reabsorbs the tissue and the pain goes away—no operation needed.

I think about these skills a lot because, like many doctors, I have the fantasy that someday I'm going to take whatever skills I have and go practice medicine somewhere in the world where they really need me. I have to warn you that this is a common doctor fantasy: When I retire, I'm joining Doctors Without Borders, I'm going on medical missions, I'm going someplace where there aren't enough doctors and see if I can really save some lives. For doctors accustomed to practicing in places like the United States, this is also the fantasy about practicing without technology, without endlessly available sophisticated imaging—x-rays and CTs and MRIs—without specialists to consult who can verify your exam, without lab tests to answer your questions. *Could I still do it without any of those things? Would I still be any use?*

After Hurricane Katrina, lots of doctors I know told themselves they should be there, not here. There were doctors who went—mostly emergency medicine special-ists, I would guess—and then there were the doctors on the spot, working in the devastated city, or caring for the displaced populations. I read the news stories about the doctors and nurses who stayed behind in the flooded hospitals, rolling the patients up to the roof so they could be airlifted out, ventilating them with bag and mask when the electricity stopped. Theirs was a particu-lar kind of heroism. They were using themselves, using what they had learned, what they had gathered profes-sionally, and they were using it against the right ene-mies—fighting the right and proper ancient battles of the medical profession against illness and infection and deterioration. In many places they were fighting them under horrifically ancient conditions.

Some of the most important, most necessary medical fields—performing heroic surgeries, providing life sup-port for the desperately ill—are the very fields most handicapped by the loss of technology; in those battles, fought out on the edge of what is possible, you need every advantage. But a great deal of the medical care that was needed after the storm was much more basic. People were sick, people were hurt, people were scared, and they needed care. Children needed their chests listened to and their asthma treated, or their skin infections man-aged with the proper antibiotics; they needed the right fluids if they were dehydrated. They needed to know they had been properly looked at and properly looked after. Even that is hard to do properly without technology so basic that we don't even notice it until it's gone.

A couple of days after the hurricane, I talked with Dr. Cindy Sheets in the pediatric clinic at the University of Alabama Children's and Women's Hospital in Mobile, Alabama, where the hospital was running on generator power. "You end up trusting more in your judgment," she said, "relying less on the backup tests you do sometimes for medicolegal reasons. Over time, you know, we all have a fair amount of experience to tell us what's going on." But the way we deliver care has come to depend extensively on technology—not just the imaging miracles of radiology and the subtleties of serology, but on the whole electronic network of communication and commerce that keeps our world turning.

Dr. Sheets was busy seeing patients, worrying about the risk of heat exhaustion to the people without power in the hot city around her. She was listening to chests and looking in ears and examining children's bodies. It wasn't even the diagnostic technology that was most on her mind. She was worried about the pharmacies: Without power, she said, many of the bigger chain pharmacies could not dispense pills or print labels. She and her colleagues were dispensing the powdered antibiotic samples they had on hand and directing patients to the few open pharmacies that were willing to compound prescriptions and provide medications without their own electric—and electronic—technological supports. She was worrying about what would happen to families after they left the clinic. Would they be able to follow the advice she had given them?

Even in the kind of relatively low-tech, relatively old-fashioned medicine I practice—primary-care pediatrics—there's an inexorable tendency to move away from relying on your own medical skills and order the extra test. Most of us know, when we train as doctors in this country, in this century, that along with our phenomenal professional arsenals—our diagnostic tests, our imaging machines, our life-support systems, our wonder drugs and even our not-quite-wonder drugs—comes a dependence on the complex web of technical support.

No one would give up the technology; we all know it helps us take better care of patients. But there is a place for legitimate regret about the skills you lose when you don't depend on them, and a place for anxiety about whether in fact, over time, you become no more than the sum of your technology. Maybe that's part of the point of the fantasy about going overseas, practicing medicine in a refugee camp, going one-on-one with disease just like in the old days. When I trained, back in what now look like the relatively low-tech 1980s, plenty of the senior doctors pointed out to us, with a bit of regret, that the art of physical diagnosis, for so many years the great point of professional pride, was being abandoned for the science of technology. They worried that those skills would be lost, in an era when you could easily obtain sophisticated images of the heart and its blood flow, when technology could answer every question you had thought to ask, resolve every diagnostic ambiguity. We were reminded over and over that there were pitfalls in trusting the technology, and I had teachers who made a special teaching point of every case where too much reliance on diagnostic tests led to wrong treatment or overtreatment or missed diagnoses. What about the guy who came to the emergency room for GI problems and told the ER doc he had a history of heart problems since he was born, though he couldn't remember the details, and they called someone in to do an echocardiogram, and imagine how embarrassing it was when they couldn't find the guy's heart right away. It turns out his heart problem was situs inversus—his heart is on the right side instead of the left—which someone would have known immediately if anyone had listened to his chest carefully with a stethoscope! Did you hear about that poor old lady who got a mega-workup for these mysterious blood infections she kept getting, and it turned out no one had looked carefully at her feet, and all along, she had this terrible open sore between her toes that was probably serving as a portal of entry for bacteria! . . . It's still a teaching truism, a reminder of the medical ironies in our technology-rich practice: "When all else fails, look at the patient."

Here's one more hurricane story—or one more story about how technology now shapes our patient care. Dr. Marsha Raulerson, a pediatrician in rural Alabama, remembers vividly when Hurricane Ivan devastated the small town of Brewton. Practicing in a rural area, she said, she probably relies less on technology than many other doctors—"I depend on my physical exam, not an x-ray," she told me—but she was devastated by the realization that she was truly and profoundly out of touch:

> *I'm always with my cell phone, I'm always with my beeper. They wouldn't work, phone lines were down. My husband said I lost my mind, I was just frantic. I ended up the day after the storm going to the office just sitting there in the dark, wondering if people were going to find me. A few wandered in, children injured during the storm, but I was just worried that if they needed help they wouldn't be able to call or to get there, so I was sending out people to check on all my high-risk babies that were at home.*

That was her biggest anxiety—not that she would have trouble diagnosing an illness, even if she was armed only with her five senses, her stethoscope, and her clinical experience. We reach our patients today through technological tools in almost every sense—we depend on their power for diagnosis and for visualization and even for conversation. But the goal and the impulse remain unchanged: The doctor in the hurricane-ravaged town was frantic because she needed to be able to touch those patients, hear their voices, let them know she was still there for them. There are many kinds of heroism, and even many kinds of medical heroism. There is the true drama of what is actually called heroic surgery—high-stakes high-tech life and death. But there is also the everyday one-on-one heroism of truly looking at the patient, listening to the patient, and carefully touching the patient, even when you're both in semidarkness.

It's easy to kid yourself—or lie to yourself or to other people—about your physical diagnosis skills. When you're in training, the desire to find "pathology" is strong, precisely because you know this is your chance to learn how to recognize the calling cards of different diseases. This is why you get into those notorious hospital situations where a patient has an "interesting physical finding" and sits there in bed facing a string of medical students and residents who have been sent into the room to learn. This isn't fun for the patient even when the physical finding is easily accessible and not particularly tender—an unusual facial tumor, let's say—but think how not fun it is for the patient if it's an unusual stomach mass that was maybe slightly tender at the beginning of the day, and has now been laboriously examined by four or five or six relative newbies. (Yes, we try not to be too insensitive about this kind of thing, and yet, how else is a medical student going to be able to build up a personal reference library of abdominal masses? Don't you want the doctor who examines you—or your child or your parent—ten years from now to have had that experience, to carry that personal reference library?)

So medical students, and residents, and even doctors wander through the hospital and through the world consciously trying to add to that index of physical diagnoses. Yes, I've heard this, yes, I've seen this, yes, I've felt this. I've palpated an enlarged liver, I've elicited an abnormal reflex with my little rubber hammer, I've noted the tremor of Parkinson's disease, I've heard the galloping heart sounds of congestive heart failure, I've looked at the back of a patient's eye and seen the abnormal blood vessels of severe hypertension, I've examined a newborn's hips and felt the click of dysplasia. All of these observations are routine, in a certain sense. They are things you look for every day when you take care of patients—we haven't even gotten to the list of the exotic diagnoses.

I can remember children being admitted to the hospital with what are now rare and interesting conditions, at least in the developed world—a kid with measles, a baby with whooping cough, an adolescent from Asia with a withered leg after polio. Every single medical student and resident was sent to check out that kid and learn what the rash of measles looked like—the real thing, not a photo—and to stand outside the room and wait for that baby's astonishing coughing spells, and to look at that adolescent's shriveled limb. There was a certain irony in sending out an all-points bulletin for people to come look at these "exotic" illnesses, which presumably all their grandmothers and great-grandmothers could have identified easily. (These examples—measles, whooping cough, polio—should make us think with great reverence about the miracles of immunization, but we'll get to that later on.) When I say to residents or medical students, when you hear the whoop of whooping cough, you'll know—it's not like anything else—I mean it, and I know what I'm talking about, but that's because I've heard it, the real thing, coming out of a real and suffering child, and not just a teaching videotape.

Or take chicken pox. When I was growing up, everyone had chicken pox. I had it, and I gave it to my younger brother, just the way you're supposed to. And you had chicken pox, Orlando, because you were born in 1984, and you promptly passed it on to your sister, who wasn't immunized either, because she was born in 1989. So you both had chicken pox in the same time-honored way, and I don't think I even called the doctor, any more than my own mother did. It was just chicken pox; you put lotion on the pox and tried to stop the child from scratching (I remember being put to bed in little white gloves, back in the early 1960s), and you treated the fever and you waited for it to go away. Certainly, you didn't need any help in making the diagnosis. (In fact, because varicella, the virus that causes chicken pox, is wildly contagious, doctors actively tried to discourage parents from bringing those children in unless they were truly unusually sick. One child with varicella in the waiting room could infect dozens, and a child on the hospital ward with varicella was the recurring infection-control nightmare of my years as a pediatric infectious diseases fellow.)

But your younger brother was born in 1995, and by the time he was a year old, we were vaccinating against chicken pox, so he's never had it. Over the past ten years, chicken pox has become pretty rare. So today, when there's a child in the clinic with the classic rash, yes indeed, I send in all the medical students (who have all had to provide documentation that they are themselves immune, either because they had the disease or because they've had the vaccine), and I stand there and point out the features, just as if it were some exotic rare condition. "Dewdrop on a rose petal," I say, over and over, describing the rash of varicella—a small vesicle containing clear fluid on a bright red base. "Lesions at different stages," I point out, because normally with chicken pox, new pox keep appearing and evolving—from red spot to bump to dewdrop on a rose petal to crusting over. And the students look closely at the itchy, spotted child, filing away yet one more important piece of arcane medical knowledge: You won't see varicella much, but when you do see it, you damn well better know it.

Rashes, at least, are right out there on the surface, to be seen and described and classified and learned. On the inside, it's different. A good friend of mine in medical school was instructed during a rotation in OB/GYN to examine a woman carefully so he could "appreciate" her pelvic mass—and by appreciate we only mean register, describe, understand. But for my friend, this involved doing one more gynecologic exam on a woman who had already had more of them than she wanted, and he felt a little uncomfortable about that. But he knew it was important to be able to appreciate a pelvic mass, so he did it, and he did it thoroughly and carefully. But he simply couldn't find the mass, let alone appreciate it. Of course, he thought about lying, just saying to his attending, yes, I felt it, very helpful, thank you. He knew, after all, that if he told the truth, the attending would probably make him subject the patient to yet one more exam, would stand over him and drive the teaching point home, and he would feel guilty toward the patient, and ashamed in front of her, as he was put through this exercise—gynecology 101, gynecology for dummies. But he decided to tell the truth, and he said to his attending honestly, no, I couldn't feel the mass. Sure enough, the attending sat him down and reexamined the patient with him, step-by-step. My friend still couldn't find the mass, even with the attending directing his every move. So, no doubt with a great sigh, and many thoughts about how they don't make medical students like they used to, and about how physical diagnosis is a lost art, the attending himself reexamined the long-suffering patient. And he couldn't find the now-famous mass.

It turned out that it was a large cyst, which had spontaneously resolved, eliminating the need for the planned surgery. The attending, to his credit, congratulated my friend, praising him for his excellent physical diagnosis skills, and also for his honesty. The attending understood perfectly the temptation to agree with the established diagnosis and confirm the received wisdom. My friend, suddenly elevated by both the doctor and the patient to a position of wisdom, skill, and experience, thanked them both for the valuable learning experience. But when he told me this story, he concluded it this way: "Little did he know, I wouldn't have been able to find the mass even if it was still there. I can never feel masses."

Natural aptitude and training and practice can make you better at feeling masses—or at listening to heart murmurs and characterizing them or at evaluating skin conditions. But it is also true that there will always be situations where two smart, well-trained doctors examine the same patient and see or hear or feel two different things. That was why the neonatology fellow was so excited to have found a mass in a newborn baby's belly—not because he was glad that the baby had a tumor, but because he was able, for the first time in his career, to trust his own fingertips to tell him that something was abnormal. That made him trust those fingertips all the other times as well, when he pronounced newborn abdomens to be normal.

There is no question that while technology makes it possible to look inside your patient, to quantify ever more obscure shadowy presences in your patient's bloodstream, it does also tend to change the way you look—or do not look—at your patient. You trust your own eyes and ears a little less, you look for confirmation before you act, you ask clinical questions partly because you know they can be answered and you want to "document" the answers. So yes, for example, "pneumonia is a clinical diagnosis," as one punctiliously reminds the residents and medical students, and yes, this is supposed to mean that if you listen with your stethoscope and hear pneumonia in a patient's chest, you treat it, no chest x-ray necessary. But in fact I often end up "questioning a pneumonia" and getting the chest x-ray and letting that guide me. Sometimes it's uncertainty—did I really hear what I think I heard? And sometimes it's that medicolegal desire to tick off every box—suppose the patient gets sicker, could I really justify *not* having gotten an x-ray? And sometimes, I confess, it's just the awareness that the x-ray is possible, the x-ray is there, the x-ray is easy.

In the end, here's what I need to tell you about the physical exam. You will learn to do it first in an embarrassed, ritualized way. You will learn the laborious, careful, inch-by-inch physical exam that a medical student does before writing up an endless system-by-system note.

You will learn how to do the pressed-for-time physical exam that an intern or a resident does. You will start by apologizing for everything you do, and then probably you will begin to feel entitled to do it. But I hope that you will always remember a little of the embarrassment and a little of the sense of wonder that people trust you with their bodies, even their sore and painful bodies, trust your touch and your probing, and allow you to pass this boundary. Perhaps, too, you will become expert in some particular piece of the physical exam. I look with awe at the assurance of good dermatologists who speak with real confidence about all the peculiar things that show up on the human skin; I marvel at what a good ophthalmologist can see by looking at the eye.

But before you ever get there, you will become experienced and matter-of-fact about all the most highly private and highly charged parts of the physical; you will walk into so many rooms and examine so many strangers, you will inspect their skin and listen to their hearts and lungs and feel all over their bodies looking for lymph nodes and lumps, you will do female genital exams and male genital exams and rectal exams—and all of this will somehow change your familiarity with the human body, your sense of privacy, and your understanding of what we all—every one of us—carry around underneath our clothing.

A couple of years ago, I went with a friend to see a performance of the play *The Vagina Monologues* when it came through Boston. She's also a pediatrician, and she specializes in teenage girls, which means she does a great deal of gynecology. We managed to get tickets at the last minute (some had been returned), and we jubilantly hurried down the aisle, found our seats, and settled down. Just as the curtain was about to go up, my friend turned and said to me, in a normal conversational tone, "So, do you think watching this show is different for people like us who actually look at vaginas all day long?" Everyone in range turned to stare at us, wondering, no doubt, about the interesting details of our lives.

I'm a pediatrician. I like examining children. I like being able to look beneath their clothing and understand what is happening to their bodies, and I like the solid reality of the physical exam. There are times when, for one reason or another, life feels out of control—the clinic is incredibly busy, the waiting room is nuts, everyone is stressed—or maybe the parent seems off the wall and the story just doesn't make sense. But it is always reassuring, or at least helpful and real, to turn to the child, to touch the child, to try to touch reassuringly and to say in words and gestures to the child and the parent, both, show me what's wrong, show me where it hurts, let's have a look.

Practicing medicine for me is completely tied up with that sense of a living body under my hands, the heart pumping and the lungs inflating and the oxygen traveling around via the blood vessels. It's life itself, with all its mysteries, and the physical exam, as you repeat it over and over again, is one of the doctor's humble ways of attempting to tease out those mysteries.

I've examined a lot of newborns by now, without ever finding that unexpected mass, and while I am grateful that it hasn't fallen to me to detect a tumor, I am also always mindful of that neonatology fellow and his excitement. Someday, I may press down on a baby's belly and feel something that no one else has detected yet, and it's my job to be ready for that.

**4**

■ The State of Residency

*Dear Orlando,*

Technically, medical school makes you into a doctor. It ends in a graduation ceremony, after all, which leaves you holding that diploma, which you will eventually frame and hang prominently on the wall. A ceremony in which you stand, together with your classmates, and recite aloud an oath—usually a version of the Hippocratic Oath, sometimes one of the newer oaths, but always a powerful statement dedicating your lives to medicine and accepting its yoke of standards, ideals, and ethics—as your parents and significant others watch in awe. You'll know an awful lot more than you did at the beginning, and you will feel that you have in some major sense crossed over into a new professional zone.

But you won't really be there yet. The most significant and transformative part of medical training is now in front of you, as residency is about to begin. The single most significant piece of all that you learned in medical school may be the choice you make in your fourth year when you apply for residency, when you sort yourself into internal medicine or orthopedic surgery or pediatrics or radiology, into dermatology or neurosurgery or family medicine.

## First: Choosing and Being Chosen

*The patient is a thirty-three-year-old woman, twenty-eight weeks pregnant, with good prenatal care, who was riding in a car that was involved in an MVA. She was in the passenger seat, wearing a seat belt; the car was stopped at a light when it was struck from behind by a small truck and crashed into another car ahead of them. She was brought to the emergency room by EMTs and was stabilized there; she has regained consciousness, although the neurosurgeons are still questioning the possibility of spinal trauma, and the surgeons are concerned about possible abdominal bleeding. However, although she consented to have limb x-rays done, she initially refused to undergo any spinal films because she is worried about x-ray exposure for the fetus. She became extremely agitated when films were suggested. She has several orthopedic fractures, one of which will require surgical repair. Meanwhile, she has been found to be in active labor, and the fetal heart tracing is showing severe distress, so the decision has been*

> *made to deliver her baby by emergency cesarean section and to repair her fracture during the same procedure, after which she will have a full series of spinal films.*

•

This vignette, based on a case I remember vividly from my medical student days, could be a novel. An MVA (motor vehicle accident), a pregnant woman with excellent prenatal care, who had done everything possible to take proper care of her unborn child, wakes up dazed in an emergency room to realize that the world had crashed in on her. And then sudden galloping active labor, probably because of the abdominal trauma and shock, and then the evidence that the fetus was in severe distress, which suddenly meant that everything had to happen in superfast time. No time to convince her to go for spinal films, no time to *do* spinal films— she would have to have her cesarean section done while she was still in the c-spine collar, which the EMTs had fastened around her neck when they pulled her from the wrecked car.

The story involved several different groups of doctors and a major coordinated effort—the ob-gyns who would deliver the baby, the orthopedic surgeons who would repair the fracture, the general surgeons who would scrub in to be there if it turned out there was more abdominal trauma and bleeding, and the neurosurgeons who were hovering in the background, in case, when all was said and done, there was in fact a spinal cord injury to repair.

I was a medical student on one of the surgical services—I think it was general surgery, though it might have been orthopedics—and everyone on my team wanted to be sure that I understood what a complicated case this was, what a challenge to everyone's expertise. This saga felt weirdly like a staged drama—we could have been doctors on TV, acting out one of those baroque scenarios that would never happen in real life. Yet those scenarios do happen all the time in the hospital, and real lives are always at stake.

This case made a tremendous impression on me, for its pathos, for its ironies. I had recently been through my own first pregnancy, and I found myself thinking about the ways pregnant women worry. In my childbirth class, women had talked about never taking even a sip of wine (to avoid any risk of fetal alcohol syndrome), about moving out of the house when renovations were under way (to avoid any possible exposure to lead dust), about never emptying the cat litter box (to avoid exposure to a parasite called *Toxoplasma gondii*, which is found in cat feces and can be dangerous to the developing fetus). I thought about the ways we take scrupulous care to protect against even rare and unlikely dangers—and then, in spite of all our precautions, come the accidents and the crashes that show us the terrifying fragility of life. The scene in the operating room felt to me like a profound professional drama: teams of different doctors and nurses, all up against unusual conditions and serious odds.

Are you surprised that I can't remember which team of surgeons I belonged to? Can you guess why not? I do remember hanging around in the operating room, trying to keep out of the way. I was interested in the dramatic story, and I appreciated the skill and speed with which the operating room team performed that cesarean section, driven by the frantic fear that the fetus might be suffering oxygen deprivation, might be suffering brain injury, and the knowledge that every minute counted. Two obstetricians worked across that woman's hardly swollen abdomen (a normal full-term pregnancy lasts forty weeks, so this woman was three full months from her due date), assisted by nurses who knew what to hand them before they even asked for it; it was as choreographed and intense as any dance of life and death could be. But as soon as they had done the C-section—and an emergency C-section happens fast, believe me—there was a second patient in the room who was handed over to yet another team of doctors, the pediatricians, who had been called over from the newborn intensive care unit. As soon as that second patient arrived, weighing all of about two pounds, I found myself hovering behind the doctors who were taking care of him. The baby was the patient who drew me, and what I wanted to learn— even though I was on the wrong rotation for it that month—was what you did with a baby born twelve weeks premature, after severe trauma to the mother.

This is a cliché about pediatricians: You find out where you belong professionally when you do your OB rotation and you discover that every time you witness the miracle of birth, you lose interest in the woman who is supposed to be your patient and you long to follow the baby. I certainly felt that way. I enjoyed taking care of the mothers, but to me they were not nearly as fascinating as their infants. I don't mean that I wanted to coo over their babies and cuddle them. I wanted to be there evaluating their distress and making the judgments about giving medications or doing CPR or checking them over for congenital anomalies. I wanted them to be my patients, I wanted to be their doctor.

Recently, I was talking with a group of first-year medical students who were lamenting their uncertainty about their future plans. Would they go into internal medicine? Would they pursue surgery? What were they really good at? Where did they belong? And one of them asked me, did you always want to be a pediatrician? No, I said honestly, I didn't know what I wanted to be. I guess that if I had given it any thought, I assumed I would go into internal medicine and concentrate on infectious diseases; that was my strongest intellectual interest. But then I started my clinical rotations, and the first one I did was internal medicine, which was also the longest and in some sense the most important of the basic rotations. To my surprise, I didn't like it at all.

I should explain that as you go through the first two years of medical school, doing your basic science coursework and studying pathophysiology, you are constantly longing for the hospital. Even if the school goes to great trouble to offer you a certain amount of patient contact, there's still the sense that real clinical medicine is just out of reach. You want to be on the wards, you want to be remembering your gross anatomy while standing in an operating room, you want to be putting your pathophysiology to use talking about patients. That's what it's all about. So when I found myself, finally, on the wards, and I didn't love it, I was dismayed. Why did I hate to get up in the morning? Why did I dread hearing that there was a patient assigned to me? Why was I tearful and oversensitive to criticism? Why did I have so much trouble learning new information and remembering what I learned? Had I made a terrible mistake in going to medical school?

Despite these feelings, I managed to work my way through the three months of internal medicine, unhappy and exhausted, puzzled and angry at myself. I had plenty of classmates who were ecstatic to be on the wards, who were finding all the challenge and all the learning they had expected, who were building strong connections with patients and consciously modeling themselves on the doctors with whom they were working. I could not understand them at all—until I started my pediatrics rotation.

Suddenly I was delighted to hear there was a patient in the ER for me to work up. And suddenly I didn't mind reading up on my patients and presenting them to the group. In fact, twenty-some years later, I still remember some of the cases from my first pediatric rotation: a girl with intractable seizures whose physician was trying a special ketogenic diet to control her epilepsy; a teenager who had taken an overdose of aspirin—probably a much less likely drug for someone to choose today, but back then a common painkiller that was in every medicine chest. And I remember them because for the first time in medical school, I had truly entered into the process of learning clinically. I wanted to understand each patient I cared for, and I wanted to remember them, and I wished I knew enough to be in charge. That extra interest and motivation came across to the residents I worked with; I was a much better medical student in pediatrics than I had been in internal medicine. I hadn't gone to medical school planning to be a pediatrician, but a pediatrician was clearly what I would become.

The lesson here is, don't get too fixed on any subspecialty before you've had a chance to try them all out. One student in my medical school class was sure he would become an intensely academic subspecialist in internal medicine—a hematologist-oncologist or a nephrologist—but he was so swept away by the challenge and the drama of psychiatry that he found himself explaining to his surprised family that psychiatry was the only place he could imagine himself. There were people who had never thought of themselves as surgeons who lit up with joy in the operating room, and there were people who had been waiting and waiting to get into the operating room who found themselves there, under the special lights, feeling distinctly, well, bored.

Orlando, you can be anything you want to be. You can be that academic gastroenterologist, or that psychiatrist, or that pediatric neurosurgeon. You think you want to be a surgeon, and it's possible that desire will last, that you will always be thrilled to walk into an operating room and solve the problems that surgery will set for you. On the other hand, you may find that surgery isn't what you expected, or that some other field pulls you even harder.

If that happens, don't be disappointed in yourself, and don't put up too much of a fight. You want to go into a field you love. You want to be a surgeon if you really understand why surgeons would rather be in the operating room than anywhere else. You want to be in the emergency room if you are truly excited to see what will roll through the door next. You want to be in primary care if you crave a role in the lifelong evolving medical stories of your patients. You will know it when you find what seem to you your right and proper problems, your right and proper patients, your right and proper colleagues. You may find that several different fields draw you, but you will definitely know when you are being drawn.

It is an amazing privilege, all your life, to know that you have found the proper fit. Finding the proper fit in medicine involves more than choosing the right specialty; you need to find the right place to train and the right setting in which to work, and you need to shape your life. When you choose internal medicine, radiology, emergency medicine, surgery, or another specialty, you are choosing a residency, but you are also choosing the intellectual and professional architecture of your career. You are selecting a set of problems that will be the problems that will engage you all your life, and you are choosing a set of patients and a group of colleagues. That knowledge will guide you into "the match." During your fourth year of medical school, you will interview at multiple residency programs in your chosen field, and you will submit a rank list. Your rank list and the rank list of every other fourth-year medical student in the country will go into the national match. Each residency program will also submit a rank list, ordering the applicants to that program, and the Great Computer in the Sky will sort you all out so you're placed in the program that ranks highest on your list, which also ranked you on their list. It's quite a process, the Match. Every fourth-year medical student submits a list, couples matching together for programs in the same city, every residency program in every field "filling" at the same computer-controlled moment. And the day the results come is treated as a ceremonial occasion, in most medical schools, a rite of passage. You will find out your fate on Match Day, in the spring, together with all your classmates and with the whole country, and then, by the beginning of July, you will be ready to start your residency.

## Next: The Eighty-Hour Week

*The patient is an eighteen-year-old white female brought to the emergency room with high fever. She was in her usual state of good health until yesterday when she developed high fever and shaking chills, which have worsened over the course of the day. She takes antidepressants. She denies any recent travel or unusual foods. Overnight in the hospital, she developed progressively higher fever and agitation, and was treated with antipyretics and tranquilizers, including Demerol. Her fever continued to climb to 107, and she went into cardiopulmonary arrest and died. Her father is now suing the hospital, claiming that mistakes with regard to possible fatal drug interactions were made by insufficiently trained and insufficiently supervised interns and residents, and that the whole medical training system is responsible for what should have been a completely preventable death.*

•

Orlando, you probably don't recognize that case, but it's one that will have a major impact on your medical training and on your life for years to come. That's the outline of the Libby Zion story, a tragedy that took place when I was a medical student, and a legal case that dragged on for years after that. Libby Zion was an eighteen-year-old college freshman in 1984; she developed a mysterious illness, and her family brought her to New York Hospital. Their regular doctor was available by phone, but she was basically taken care of by the residents overnight, because that's who was in the hospital. During the night, she got sicker and died. And indeed, her father, Sidney Zion, who is a well-known journalist, did sue the hospital. It was a complicated case, because there was no clear cause of death, but she had been given one medication, Demerol, that could have rare serious interactions with the antidepressant she had been taking. As I recall, there was confusion: What had she told which doctor about what medications she was taking? Had she really been given enough Demerol to cause this deadly reaction? Was there evidence that the Demerol combined with a medication she was taking was what had killed her? What *had* actually killed her?

The lawsuit involved the strange calculus of medical malpractice. Initially, a jury found that the doctors had indeed made mistakes, but held that she herself was 50 percent responsible for her own death, because she had possibly ingested cocaine (this was the hospital's claim; they were clearly trying to establish that she had caused her own death, either by taking drugs or by not telling the doctors what drugs she had taken). Her father pursued the case past that initial judgment, furiously trying to "clear her name," and finally, in 1995, eleven years after her death, the judge set aside that part of the verdict—that she was 50 percent responsible—but at the same time, reduced the financial award to her parents by half.

When I was doing my residency, I remember reading—somewhat obsessively—the accounts of the care that Libby Zion had received, asking myself over and over, would I have done anything differently? Would I have looked up the medications I was prescribing more conscientiously than her intern did? Would I have consulted with other doctors before giving her a dose of a drug I thought I was familiar with? No intern could read these stories without getting that there-but-for-the-grace-of-god feeling in the pit of the stomach. But there was another reason that any intern, back in the 1980s, would have felt particularly vulnerable: whatever the real cause of death, there was no question that this unfortunate young woman had spent her last night alive without ever being checked by a senior, experienced doctor. She had been cared for by an intern—"eight months out of medical school," echoed every news story—but an intern couldn't be much more than eight months out of medical school—by the time you're a year out of medical school, you're done with internship. And the intern had been supervised by a junior resident, one year further along (of course), both of them working long shifts (of course) and sleep-deprived (of course) and responsible for many sick patients (of course). And so, since *I* was at the time not long out of medical school, and since *I* spent many nights in the hospital sleep-deprived and worrying about sick patients, I worried that *I* might hurt someone. A book that was later published on the case was subtitled *Every Patient's Nightmare*, but it seemed to me also every intern's nightmare.

The Libby Zion case turned into something much more than an individual lawsuit about mistakes that had or had not been made late at night in an individual hospital. Sidney Zion had blamed the medical system for his daughter's death, and it became a case that changed the medical system. The State of New York convened a commission to study the hours residents worked, and in 1989, just as my residency was ending, we heard that the Bell Commission was going to limit residents to working eighty hours a week, instead of the hundred-plus hours that we all routinely worked. We shook our heads over it. Would it really happen? Would it really be enforced? Who would take care of the patients?

In fact, enforcement of those Bell Commission rules in the State of New York was apparently hit or miss. But then in 2003, the American College of Graduate Medical Education, the agency that accredits residency programs, implemented similar rules: no residents to work more than eighty hours a week. No one to work more than twenty-four hours at a stretch. No discretion for the programs; if a resident has maxed out his hours, he must be sent home or the program will be penalized. Those rules govern medical training today. I don't think anyone would claim that they are always followed absolutely, but every program tries to work with them, tracking resident hours, setting up cross-coverage systems so that people can sign out their patients and go home, scheduling in "night float" residents who come on at night and take care of patients so their colleagues can get some sleep.

I don't know whether these changes would have kept Libby Zion alive, but they are in many ways the long-overdue commonsense regulation that the medical profession needed. Everyone knows that truck drivers and airline pilots aren't allowed to take the controls if they've been working for too many hours straight. In fact, truck drivers are required to keep official sleep logs; no one wants overtired bleary-eyed drivers out on the road, speeding along in those eighteen-wheelers. So why would you allow overtired young doctors to treat patients in the hospital? To calculate their drug dosages and manage the complex life-support equipment that beeps and hums today in every ICU? Why would you let someone who has only slept for two hours of the previous twenty-four perform surgery?

So the residency world has changed, at least a little. There are probably still lots of programs (especially surgical training programs) that bend the rules, but there are rules today and everyone knows it. You are supposed to sign out and go home early after you have worked all night, even if you're absorbed in something and eager to stay (and insisting that you got plenty of sleep, thanks to the night float). When I was a resident, there were no rules, and there was no expectation at all that you would go home early, and there was no such thing as sending home a resident who was willing to stay and work longer.

It's something of an occupational disease in medicine to ramble on about what things were like back in the old days (also known as "the good old days," also known as "the days of the giants," also known as "when I was a resident"). I heard plenty of lectures on this subject during my residency, and you'll hear them too, and I apologize, as your mother, for contributing to this chorus, because I remember clearly how irritating it was to be working harder than I had ever worked in my life, and then to have to listen to people talk about how easy I and the other residents had it, compared to the good old days. Sometimes the principle of the story is how hard we worked: we weren't like you spoiled crybabies today; we worked a hundred hours, a hundred and twenty hours, a hundred and forty hours a week. Oh yeah? Well, in my program, *we* worked *two* hundred hours a week! (Wait a minute, there aren't two hundred hours in a week, but never mind.) And there were all those other things we did that you ungrateful spoiled children today never have to do—we centrifuged our own urine, did our own cell counts on spinal fluid, plated our own bacterial cultures. We didn't have the lab—or the phlebotomists or the IV team—holding our hands and doing our jobs for us. Most of all, though, we didn't have anyone supervising us. Especially at night and on weekends, when all the senior doctors went home, and the residents basically ran the hospital.

People sometimes ask, can you really work a hundred, or a hundred and twenty hours a week? Sure, here's how it works: You're on call Monday, so you work from eight a.m. Monday right through the night and then all the next day (remember, we're talking about the bad old days). Let's say they get you out at six p.m., because they feel sorry for you because you're post-call. That's thirty-four hours, now go home and sleep. But be back the next morning, Wednesday, and work from eight to eight. So we're up to forty-six hours, and look, it's Thursday morning, and you're on call again—this is an every-third-night rotation. So Thursday and Thursday night and all day Friday give you another thirty-four hours, and here we are at our eighty. But hospitals need coverage on the weekend as well. Let's say this particular program gives you Sundays off if you aren't on call, but—guess what—you're on call again! So if you worked your usual twelve hours on Saturday and then came in Sunday morning and worked for twenty-four hours, well, by Monday morning your week's total would be 116. Mind you, there might be times you had to come in well before eight a.m., and days you didn't get to go home as early as eight p.m. And there were surgical residencies in which call was every other night and not every third night. So yes, it can be done. It's painful and debilitating and harsh, but it can be done.

It's a good thing, right, that today they can't make you do it. The accrediting agencies are probably right not to leave it to the hospital's discretion. People my age and older might have great difficulty sending a resident home if we didn't have to. Some of that may be the punitive effects of our own training—if we had to put up with this, then you have to put up with this—but more of it is probably that in order to work those hours, we had to absorb a certain ethos of responsibility and continuity of care. In other words, one of the ways you made it through the pain was to tell yourself that it was important for your patients that you stayed in the hospital all those hours and took responsibility for their care, and one of the ways you made it through the fatigue was to tell yourself that damn it all, at least you were learning—

and in fact there was no other way to learn what you had to learn. You had to watch as patients evolved from hour to hour, you had to feel that you were the one on the line so that you could gather the information you needed, you had to make decisions and stay there in the hospital to see the results. I'm afraid that for many of us, those attitudes are so profoundly part of how we think about residency that it can be hard for us to contemplate sending residents home early without worrying that it will either hurt patient care or hurt resident education.

As your mother, I am deeply grateful that you will never have to wander through the hospital in the dangerous daze that comes at the end of a sleepless thirty-six-hour shift. It's a good and long-overdue phenomenon that the medical profession should regulate hours and apply those basic truck driver standards to medical residency.

But I must warn you, there are problems. They aren't necessarily insoluble, but they haven't really been solved. First, supervision is still an issue. You are unlikely to be left as completely on your own as people my age were often left; your training program will have stricter rules about more senior doctors being available in the hospital and by phone. Attending physicians really do work harder than they used to in teaching hospitals; they see the patients more regularly, write in the charts in more detail. They were always the nominal authorities, but back when I was a resident, it was clear that many of them didn't want to hear about the details of patient management—and now they do. That is without question better for the patients, because there used to be not enough supervision, and there used to be so much pressure not to call for help.

When I was doing that internal medicine rotation, the one I didn't like, I was paired with an intern on her on-call nights. It was July and she was terrified—brand-new at this, working in a competitive residency program, taking care of very sick patients. Over and over, she told me that to ask for help during the night was a sign of weakness. It was her job to figure out what to do with the patients, not to ask anyone (like a junior resident, who had already been doing this job for a year, let alone an attending) for anything. She was perfectly serious, and probably she was absolutely right about the culture of her hospital and her residency program: They *would* think she was weak if she asked for help. That was the word, weak. It gave me the creeps way back then, and it gives me the creeps to think about it now.

I hope you'll always have good supervision as you train—someone who can teach you what you need to know and step in so that your inexperience never hurts a patient. On the other hand, too much supervision and too much hand-holding, and you'll be a senior resident who has never really felt in charge—and that's not good for your future patients either. I know that you will still need—as every resident has always needed and will always need—to move toward taking full responsibility, to feel yourself able to manage progressively more complicated situations and sicker patients on your own. I hope that by the time you're doing your residency, we'll all be that much better at helping you take those necessary steps while providing you with the backup and supervision you need. And I hope you never hear the word *weak* used on a hospital ward except with reference to a patient's muscle tone.

But back to work-hour reform. There's a big issue about continuity of care and cross-coverage. When I think back about residency, I have all kinds of memories connected to working hours. I can clearly remember what it felt like to stay late on a post-call day, to be stuck in the hospital as your thirty-sixth hour ticked away, your eyelids grainy and your hands starting to shake a little, either from fatigue or from excess Diet Coke consumption. I can remember asking another intern to double-check my calculations when it came time to adjust drug dosages, because I just didn't trust my tired brain, and I can remember other interns asking me the same favor. Everyone understood that weird, awful post-call state; we'd all been there and back again. I can remember yearning to slip away to the tiny claustrophobic call room, to stretch out in my scrubs on the mattress and sink immediately into an uneasy waiting-to-be-paged kind of sleep. I can remember that beeper going off, and the sense of resenting my patients (sick, helpless children!) because they generated fevers or lost their IV lines late at night, and therefore, it seemed to me, deliberately and maliciously disturbed my sleep. I can remember sneaking off to call home and apologize because even though I had already been away all day, all night, and all day, still I wouldn't be able to leave for a while yet. There were too many sick kids, or there was one very sick kid, or there had been some kind of emergency—and I can remember feeling on the verge of tears because no matter what I did, I would be in the wrong, with my hospital team, with my patients, with my family. I learned, among other things, that you can't trust your own emotional judgment when you're that tired or that overworked; you burst into tears or bite people's heads off, you feel sorry for yourself or angry at innocent bystanders.

But there are other kinds of memories. I remember a friend of mine talking on the phone with her husband. It was his birthday, and she had made special arrangements to sign out early (like at six p.m.) so she could go out to dinner with him and have a special evening to make up for all the evenings she was gone. He was outside the hospital in his car, waiting for her. But a child she had been taking care of for weeks had suddenly gotten frighteningly sick, and she just didn't feel she could leave. So she was on the phone with him, saying helplessly, you know I wouldn't do this if it were just an ordinary thing. What she didn't want to say was that she was afraid that this child, who had been sick with a rare disease for a long time, had just undergone some kind of catastrophic neurological change—that he might be suddenly and shockingly dying—and that if this news had to be given to his family, she needed to be there to give it. I remember that after she spoke to her husband, she and I had a brief conversation about how impossible it was to convey this feeling to someone not a doctor, someone who had never done a residency. If she had been telling the story to another pediatric intern, she would just have said, my longtime patient with a chronic immunosuppressive disease apparently had some kind of major neurologic event and we don't know which way he's going. But how could her husband, sitting outside in the car, be expected to understand? I remember patients of my own who kept me awake all night and worried all the next day, children who seemed to me so complex that no one else could possibly understand them.

When a patient was *mine*—when I admitted the child, saw what the child looked like coming in to the hospital, took part in sorting out all the data and making the plan, cared for that child over the first day and night in the hospital—well, I really knew that patient, I felt responsible for that patient, and I felt that the family really knew me. To them, I was the face of the hospital—or so I believed—the person who had been there with them from the very beginning of the admission. Am I saying that today that sense of commitment and long-term involvement is gone? No, not at all. The residents I see today are driven by the same strong professional and personal imperatives. Residency is intense and overwhelming and you do your best. Sometimes no matter what you do, the outcome isn't good, and you have to learn to deal with that. But the residents today have so much signing out to do, and so much cross-coverage. They are in the hospital somewhat less, and a great deal of their time and energy is spent on signing people out. It sometimes seems they find themselves too overburdened cross-covering large numbers of patients they hardly know. So in the middle of the night—or even in the early evening—patients can easily find themselves in a hospital staffed largely by residents who may be somewhat less sleep-deprived than in past years, but who may also be profoundly stressed taking care of huge numbers of patients so their colleagues can be home getting their mandated sleep.

So that's another problem we have to solve. What happened is the officials reduced the hours without reducing the patient load—because how can you reduce the patient load? Residents have to be sent home when their shifts are up, no matter how many patients are already on the ward, no matter how many admissions are coming into the emergency room, no matter how sick some of those patients may be.

## Always: Real Life, Real Death

*The patient is an eighty-five-year-old female with severe insulin-dependent diabetes of many years standing, which has damaged her kidneys and left her blind. She also has a history of hypertension and heart disease. She lives in senior citizen housing, with an aide who comes to take care of her every day. Three days ago, the aide found her unresponsive in her bed, and she was brought to the hospital, where a CT scan revealed a massive stroke. She has continued to require mechanical ventilation to maintain good oxygen levels and has not been responsive to external stimuli. A family conference has been arranged to discuss end-of-life decision making.*

A couple of years ago, I accompanied my mother and my cousins to a hospital in Brooklyn where my aunt was dying. She had had a massive stroke, and her family had met with the neurologist and made the decision to discontinue extreme measures. In other words, they wanted her to be taken off the ventilator, but they wanted her to be left in peace, and they wanted to stay with her. I have to say that all day the care at this hospital had seemed terrific. Wonderful doctors had spent time with my family, explained the issues, discussed the options. Everyone had agreed on the parameters—pain medications, comfort, private room, no needles, no breathing tube, peace and quiet. They were sensitive and understanding, those doctors, and they paid proper attention to the sad ending of a life.

But now it was evening, and all those doctors were gone. I was trying to find someone who could order pain medication because my aunt seemed uncomfortable. I stood at the nurses' station, while the nurse paged first one intern and then another. She had a sheet detailing the night coverage that was the most complicated such sheet I had ever seen, and she herself seemed unable to decipher it. Even the page operator didn't seem to be sure who was covering. Meanwhile, I was trying to pull rank: I'm a physician, I said; I know whereof I speak, I need you to find me the intern who's covering so we can get an order written for morphine. The subtext was, I'm a physician, I'm watching you, I'm judging you, I know how serious a dereliction it is if you can't find me a responsible doctor.

Some interns answered the pages but said that this particular ward—or this particular patient—was not part of their cross-coverage responsibilities. There were some interns who didn't answer—presumably the ones who had signed out and left. Finally we found the correct cross-covering intern. He showed up with a clipboard full of sign-out notes, and spent a while going through them until he located my aunt. Of course, she was a patient he had never seen or examined, and she had probably gotten short shrift when the residents were signing out, since she was a patient for whom he was not expected to do anything. His head was full of worries—and his clipboard full of notes—about the critically ill and worrisome patients, about people who needed their respiratory difficulties and their fevers and their urinary outputs assessed and treated. And here I was, nagging him to do something for a woman who was not expected to live out the night. I could see by watching him that I was being a major pain in the ass. But he did his best for me; he looked at my aunt's chart and checked the clipboard on which the nurses were recording her vital signs and verified that all the legal papers had been signed—and he ordered the morphine. But he also apparently gave the nurse a verbal order to start an IV and give her fluids, and so a little later, there I was, paging him again, telling him that her children did not want my aunt to get an IV, they didn't want any extra needles, they didn't want any medical apparatus in the room with her. The intern, barely able to control his impatience by this point, told me that her blood pressure was a little low, probably because she was dry, and he wanted to give her some normal saline. So I went through it all again—she's dying, why do we need to improve her blood pressure?

He was probably a reasonable guy. He wanted to do the right thing. He didn't want to make a mistake. But he had no involvement in the case—he hadn't played any part in those complicated, sensitive discussions. He was more or less alone on this. At that point I wished passionately that one of the doctors who had spent the day talking with us would show up—tired or not, overworked or not—someone who felt a connection to the case and the family. I had to keep biting back those pompous words about how we did things when I was a resident, back in the days of the giants.

I suggested that he call the senior resident who had been part of the family conference. But he wasn't allowed to call her; the work-hour rules mean you have to turn off your beeper when you leave. I suggested he call one of the attendings, since they are not protected by work-hour rules, but he was clearly reluctant to bother an attending over something that was not, after all, a critical management question that might make a life-or-death difference in a patient's care.

I was asking him to let the nurses go on recording low blood pressures, low urine output, without doing anything to correct them. He looked through the paper chart, and I stood over him (oh, he really appreciated having me there, I could tell) and pointed out everything that had been signed. I'm a physician, I said to him, over and over. No IV. Look, here's where the papers were signed, by her family. Yes, said the intern, I see where it says no ventilator, no CPR—but I don't see that it says no IV. And her blood pressure is low. So we went around again.

In the end, I had it my way. I knew the language and I knew the drill. If I hadn't been a physician—and a pushy physician at that—I think it would have been hard to win this argument, and it would probably have ended up as another hospital horror story, another deathbed that was not what it should have been, more pain for the patient, more pain for the family. Even so, I would have to tell you, the doctor involved was doing his best. But there I was, a pushy physician. I told him to document our conversation clearly in the chart. I told him if he had a problem with what we were doing, I was going to have the hospital operator call the attending. While we were talking, his beeper went off six times with labs and dosage questions and sudden emergencies on other patients. He answered each page, and he said into the phone each time, wait while I look it up, I don't know this patient, I'm just cross-covering. Finally he made his note in my aunt's chart and went off to answer the next six questions, looking harried and scared, like any on-call intern.

Orlando, I know you will work hard during your residency, whatever the details of your schedule. An eighty-hour week is a serious work week. But what I hope is that you will get to feel that you know your patients, that you stay with them over time and feel fully responsible for them, that you understand the complicated family issues and the decision making. Once again, I find myself hoping that by the time you start your residency, medical education will be a little closer to making this work, to teaching residents what they need to learn, and to taking care of patients in a way that guards their safety and lets them know they have been properly noticed and known.

**5**

■ **Bugs, Drugs, and Data**

*A six-month-old infant is brought to the emergency room because her mother says she feels warm. In the exam room, the baby has a temperature of 105. You carefully look her over, but you can't find any reason for her fever—her lungs are clear and without pneumonia, her ears show no sign of an ear infection. She's cranky, but after you give her some ibuprofen and her fever comes down, she becomes calmer and drinks her bottle for a little while. What immunization question has most bearing on your decisions about how to handle this baby?*

*Dear Orlando,*

Every field in medicine has its rule-outs. A rule-out refers to the diagnosis—whatever it is—that you absolutely don't want to miss, not even once, and that you go looking for in lots of extra patients, just so you don't miss it when it really does come along. Rule out has its own abbreviation: r/o. In internal medicine, there's the need to look for a heart attack in someone who has chest pain—a rule-out MI (myocardial infarction). You would rather bring a few extra patients into the hospital, monitor them carefully, check their ECGs and their cardiac enzymes, only to conclude that they're really just having heartburn—or anxiety—or even a little extra angina. When you find that someone is not, in fact, having a heart attack, you say, "He ruled out." In surgery, think about appendicitis. "He's coming in for a rule-out appy," I would tell the emergency room when I sent in a child with bad stomach pain and vomiting. "It may just be gastroenteritis, but his belly's pretty tender." If the pain had completely gone away by the time the child was finally examined by a surgeon, or if abdominal x-rays were unconcerning and the blood tests normal, or if the patient was admitted to the hospital and watched carefully overnight and did not in fact appear to be developing appendicitis, the surgeons say, "She ruled out." Ruling out is about extra vigilance. It's about the medical mentality of always looking for the worst possible diagnosis, before you settle for the more common, less dangerous possibilities. Ruling out is about not missing anything. As an internist, you might talk to dozens of people every week about their chest pain, but if you miss the one who's really having the heart attack, what good is all that training and all that practice?

In general pediatrics, ruling out is most commonly about severe bacterial infections, also known as sepsis. The case at the beginning of this chapter would be a typical rule-out sepsis dilemma. When I was learning to be a pediatrician, admitting a child to the hospital in order to rule out bacterial sepsis was so common that we usually just called such an admission "a rule-out." That's what the emergency room would tell you when they called: "We've got a five-month-old rule-out here for you." On morning rounds after being on call, that's how you would present it—"This kid is basically admitted for a rule-out." Rule-out sepsis admissions were part of bread-and-butter pediatrics, usually routine, occasionally interesting, once in a while scary. I mean, these bugs are nasty. I was reminiscing with a friend my age about residency, and we started recalling a case—the infant who came in with fever and what looked like pneumonia, and tested positive for a virus, RSV, which often causes respiratory infections in young babies. The doctors thought they had an explanation for his fever and his generally ill appearance, and there was no need for antibiotics because it was a viral infection—and then in the middle of the night, he "crashed," as we say; he needed more and more oxygen and his blood pressure dropped and he almost died. So he was moved to the intensive care unit and treated with all kinds of drugs, including antibiotics, and a bacterium *Haemophilus influenza* grew out of everything—his blood, his urine, his lung secretions. The viral infection had been strictly a by-the-way.

The idea behind a rule-out sepsis admission is this: Babies are more vulnerable to serious bacterial infections. Their immune systems don't work perfectly, they aren't loaded up with the immunities you acquire after even a couple of years in the world, rubbing up against other children and adults, and they even have some anatomical vulnerabilities. For example, the blood-brain barrier is a little leakier in young infants; if there are bacteria in the blood, it's easier for that infection to get into the brain and the spinal cord and cause meningitis.

So I want you to imagine me, in the 1980s, a pediatric resident, called to the emergency room to see that baby in the case. A young infant—six months old. A high fever. Two anxious parents. I've looked at the baby carefully, and I can't find a source for the fever—no red eardrums to suggest an ear infection, no crackles in the lungs to point toward pneumonia. Just a little baby with a high fever. So I look in all the likely places that a hidden bacterial infection might lurk—I take a urine sample to send for culture to look for a urinary tract infection, a sample of blood to look for bacteremia, a bacterial infection of the bloodstream, and I do a spinal tap to get some cerebrospinal fluid. Way back when, my ability to do those things was part of my stock-in-trade as a resident, part of my skill set—the speed and efficiency with which I could get those little vials of fluid out of a baby, following sterile procedures, so that there would be no contaminating bacteria to confuse the issue.

So let's do it: the basic baby sepsis workup. It isn't exactly fun, especially for the baby, but it has to be done. And to tell you the truth, it *is* kind of fun for me, in a doctorly way: My job is clear, I like doing these basic procedures, and if I do them right, I'll feel a certain sense of accomplishment. So I get a nice clean urine sample by passing a catheter up the baby's urinary tract and into the bladder. Unfortunately, this baby is a girl. It's easy to catheterize a circumcised male baby—kind of a straight shot, you might say. Swab his little penis with Betadine, grip it firmly in your gloved hand, and there's the meatus, the urinary opening, and you can pass the catheter right in. On the other hand, circumcised males have a low rate of urinary tract infections—they're more likely to occur in uncircumcised males. But this is a female—and females are much more likely than any males, circumcised or not, to get these infections, because their urinary tracts are shorter and it's so easy for bacteria to travel up from the diaper. And females are just much trickier to catheterize.

But let's say I get the urine, and then I get the blood by drawing blood cultures, first swabbing the skin a couple of times with alcohol and then with disinfectant, and then injecting the blood I've drawn into special blood culture bottles, full of liquid bacterial medium. Finally I get the cerebrospinal fluid by doing a lumbar puncture—

and now I am wearing a sterile gown as well as a face mask and sterile gloves. A nurse positions this now very angry baby on her side, bending her almost double to stretch the vertebral spaces as far as possible, and I drape her with sterile sheets and swab the skin over her spinal cord with disinfectants. I carefully introduce the spinal needle through the skin and through the membranes around the spinal cord—feeling for a tiny characteristic pop—and then I hold my needle steady and let the precious spinal fluid drip out, drop by drop, into my four little sterile tubes. The fluid looks nice and clear, which is good news from two points of view. First, it doesn't look cloudy, the way spinal fluid can look if you really do have bacterial meningitis—the white cells in the spinal fluid are the hallmark of the disease. Second, since the most important quick test I'm going to do on this fluid is to look for that hallmark, I feel lucky the fluid is not contaminated with blood; that makes it much easier to get a nice unequivocal test result.

But back to our rule-out. I'm busy packaging up all my tubes for the lab—the urine goes to be checked for various substances, spun in a centrifuge, and looked at under the microscope—and most important, carefully inoculated into bacterial culture medium. So we'll watch the urine cultures and the blood cultures in their special bottles, and finally my precious tubes of cerebrospinal fluid will go to different labs—one to bacteriology, to be looked at under a microscope and inoculated into petri dishes, one to the hematology lab, where they'll count the red blood cells and the white blood cells, and one to the chemistry lab, where they'll measure the glucose and the protein. We'll get a certain amount of information back in the next couple of hours. We'll know if the urine has white blood cells in it, for example, which often signals a urinary tract infection, and we'll know about the spinal fluid glucose and protein, which, again, are abnormal if you've got meningitis. But what we won't be able to find out immediately is whether anything is going to grow in any of those bacterial cultures—urine, blood, or CSF. For all bacterial infections, you can look for clues and signs, but the absolute gold standard is to grow the bacteria.

Thus, the rule-out. The little girl is about to be admitted to the hospital and started on IV antibiotics, which she'll be on for forty-eight hours—if the cultures stay negative. In other words, she'll rule out. In two days, we'll feel we can believe she doesn't have meningitis or bacterial sepsis or even a urinary tract infection. We'll say she's ruled out—and we'll mean that her fever was probably caused by a virus, which doesn't require antibiotics, and which will get better by itself. We know, from the start, that a viral infection is statistically far more likely than the bacterial infections we're so busy ruling out. But we're sufficiently worried about the possibility of those infections that we're going to treat her until we're sure. We've all seen babies who came in sick and dying with bacterial sepsis, babies whose brains were destroyed by meningitis, and we have institutionalized this process so we don't miss one.

Maybe I got a little carried away there, taking you through that rule-out sepsis. I guess it was my chance to show you one aspect of the day-and-night substance of my residency. I wanted to bring up the idea of the rule-out to remind you that in medicine, you are always supposed to worry about the worst possible outcome. I wanted you to see what some of the specific worries were that shaped me as a pediatrician—and to see how we constructed protocols and procedures to address those worries. But I also wanted to talk about how protocols change, and about why pediatric residents no longer spend so much time doing these procedures.

The rule-out sepsis still exists in pediatrics. If you go into my field, you will still learn this drill. But you won't need to do nearly as many as I did. That's the point I wanted to make with this particular case—before I found myself wanting to take you through the workup. The question I posed was this: What immunization question has most bearing on your decisions about how to handle this baby? To answer it, we have to go beyond the technicalities of the sepsis workup and think about what I was afraid of—which bacteria was I looking for, and what harm would they do if they were there?

I want to name two bacteria in particular. *Haemophilus influenzae* type B, and *Streptococcus pneumoniae*. Or, as we call them more familiarly, H. flu and Strep pneumo. These were the real bad actors, the ones statistically most likely to cause serious bacterial infections in young children. I spent my residency in fear of H. flu meningitis. Children with H. flu meningitis often died of the overwhelming disease, but if they made it through, many of them were left deaf or brain damaged. H. flu also caused other devastating infections; as with many bacteria, it liked to invade certain parts of the body, causing certain bad syndromes. Periorbital cellulitis—a dangerous purple-tinged swelling of the skin around the eye. Epiglottitis—a rapidly progressive infection of the epiglottis, which could swell so badly that it could suddenly cut off your airway. Strep pneumo was the most common pathogen that would grow in our blood cultures—it caused serious blood infections, but it also had a propensity to invade the spinal cord and the lungs.

I spent my residency watching out warily for these bad actors, H. flu type B and Strep pneumo. Looking for them more often than I found them, ruling out kids right and left, occasionally treating the infections and noting their destructive virulence. But you and your classmates probably won't see them, and won't even worry about them much, because we now vaccinate all children against both bacteria. We started vaccinating against H. flu back when today's medical students were growing up, and we added a vaccine against Strep pneumo about six years ago. That takes those bacteria more or less out of the equation, so the right answer to the question in the clinical case is that you better ask whether that baby's immunizations are up to date. A six-month-old should have had three doses of both vaccines, and a baby who has had three doses of both vaccines is pretty well protected. In other words, we would no longer do a "routine" rule-out sepsis on such a baby.

Of course, you'd do it if the baby looked really sick. Or if the baby hadn't gotten her shots (maybe she's a new immigrant, or maybe her parents are crunchy-granola types and get their health care from an herbal practitioner who doesn't believe in immunizations), you might do the workup. I examined a baby a couple of years ago who had gotten only one set of shots by the age of eight months—because he kept getting colds and his parents didn't want him to suffer through getting shots when he was sick, and because they missed an appointment here and there. There he was, eight months old and almost unvaccinated. He had a high fever and he looked sick. Hard to console, he was clingy and fretful and a little out of it. If he had been a fully immunized eight-month-old, I would have given him some fever medicine and waited for the fever to come down. If he started to look any better, I would just have sent him home. But I sent this baby to the emergency room, with instructions to do a full sepsis workup. Even if he looks better when his fever is down, I thought, he's still unprotected. I thought about all the worst outcomes I had seen during residency. So that baby did get a full workup, and he was admitted to the hospital. Nothing grew—it was a viral infection all along. But at least they gave him his next set of shots before they sent him home.

It's remarkable to watch diseases disappear. Sometimes I feel funny about the experience and expertise that we developed but rarely use in practice anymore. Think for a minute about what it means that those diseases are gone. Think about the epidemiology that gathered the information. Think about the accumulated clinical expertise that went into managing those diseases and teaching new doctors to look for them and recognize them and manage them. Then think about the many years of research that go into developing, testing, and proving safe a new vaccine. And once the vaccine is institutionalized and given routinely and the disease starts to disappear, think about how quickly we lose sight of it as a threat.

Look around your medical school class. If there were no vaccines, there would be, among the hundred and fifty or so of you, students who would have been affected by every single one of the diseases we vaccinate against. You would all have had measles—that was an illness that everyone got back before shots. Now you may never see a patient with measles—or at least, if one does come in to the hospital, you can be sure that you'll all be sent to gawk at the unusual case. But once upon a time, you would all have had measles, and it's a miserable illness.

Horrible rash, horrible high temperatures, child feels just awful. Most of you would have recovered from the measles; a couple might have gone on to develop brain infections or serious pneumonia—or gone blind. And most of you would probably have had whooping cough—pertussis—and again, it's an awful experience, but you would have recovered—except for the ones who caught it very young and died. Then there's diphtheria. I've seen measles and I've actually had whooping cough, but I don't think I've ever seen a case of diphtheria, that severe membranous tonsillitis that can choke you to death. So there would be empty chairs in your medical school classroom from all of these—from measles, from diphtheria, from polio, which would have killed some and left others disabled. And that's before we get to the rarer serious infections I've been describing above, H. flu disease and Strep pneumo.

It's a small miracle to me that you can examine that feverish six-month-old, learn that she's had her immunizations, and decide to send her home without antibiotics, without having to worry that it's H. flu and she may be dead by morning. It's a small clinical change, but it reflects a complex web of research and policy, so you might stop to tip your hat to the army of lab researchers, bacteriologists, vaccinologists, biochemists, cell culture specialists, and geneticists who developed these vaccines, and the epidemiologists and clinical researchers who tested them and measured their effects. You might stop and tip your hat, but you won't. We come so quickly to take medical progress for granted. There's no one practicing medicine in this country who lies awake worrying about polio—or even about H. flu. In a certain sense, I think we all tend to stop believing in the diseases we don't see regularly and don't have to worry about—not just the doctors, but also the patients. That's why there are so many parents, I think, who are willing to contemplate not vaccinating their children—which, as you have probably guessed by now, is something that brings out my more irritable side.

My parents, who grew up in the 1930s, still had vivid memories of the annual polio epidemics in New York City. They would never have dreamed of skipping any kind of vaccination; the illnesses were too vivid in their memories. They knew about polio, and whooping cough, and measles. But those diseases seem more and more remote to people born in the 1970s and 1980s as they make decisions about their own children. For them the hypothetical (and, I have to tell you, often scaremongering) risks of bad side effects from a vaccine can seem much more immediate than the real devastation left by the measles virus. Why should I be surprised if parents don't want to vaccinate their children against diseases they've barely heard of and never seen? There's been so much publicity around the real (though rare) and the alleged side effects of vaccines, and there are so many terrifying stories on the Internet about perfect healthy children who became autistic—or retarded—or just dropped dead after they were vaccinated. There's been excellent research done that debunks the link between the MMR vaccine and autism, but that gets much less publicity, and it certainly doesn't make it onto those Internet antivaccine sites. There is no comparable publicity, and there are no comparable horror stories out there about the diseases themselves, about the previously healthy, delightful child left retarded or deaf or dead after measles or meningitis. So I shouldn't be surprised, and I suppose I shouldn't be angry, but I am part of that medical generation that still saw children devastated and dying from H. flu and Strep pneumo, and I am not good with parents who refuse their children this protection.

It doesn't help my native hostility that many of these parents are happy to take advantage of all the other children getting immunized—you're much less likely to get measles if all the other children in the school get their shots, so why not let your precious little darling skip the nasty needle and just ride safely on the back of the herd immunity? But as the years go by, the medical profession is increasingly asking parents to protect their children against threats that to them must seem vague and shadowy and almost quaintly historical.

Most of these diseases are not gone; they are still killing thousands and tens of thousands of people elsewhere in the world. Measles kills a half million children every year, and collectively, the vaccine-preventable diseases kill well over a million. If I have made you feel that it is a great and glorious thing that you can practice here without anticipating too many cases of these diseases, you might then ask yourself what it means about our world that these preventable diseases are killing six-month-olds on other continents.

In fact, you should probably spend some time on one of those other continents during your training. It's increasingly common for medical students or residents to do some time abroad, and it will help you understand a great deal about the choices that we make, as a society, as a country, as a world. It will also give you a chance to see all kinds of interesting diseases that you aren't likely to encounter here. As a medical student, I spent a month in London working at the Hospital for Tropical Diseases, and I got to hang out in the leprosy clinic. And I have to tell you that if you say that to a group of medical students, they will all answer, "Cool!" I also spent a month in New Delhi, which means I saw cases of tuberculous meningitis and lots of other fascinating—and, in many cases, totally preventable—diseases. But I didn't go work abroad as a resident—it wasn't as common back then—and I wish I had. I think I would understand the world a little better, and I think I would probably be a better doctor for it.

Okay, back into our little room with our hot little patient. I'll be the ghost of workups past, hovering over your shoulder, already planning how I'll lay out my needles and my tubes and my labels. You must make sure you take this child seriously—just because she's immunized is no reason to dismiss her fever and her pain. Damn it, she's only six months old, her immune system is impaired, and she's got a fever of 105—do you have any idea what that feels like? If you had a fever of 105, you'd be a miserable little puddle on the floor, moaning and groaning and feeling like death warmed over. (Babies and young children actually handle fevers somewhat better than adults; there are plenty of toddlers who are still running around and playing with a temp of 103 or 104—hence the affectionate expression, hot tots.) You better make absolutely sure she doesn't have pneumonia—listen carefully to her chest, observe her breathing, get a chest x-ray if you have any doubts. You better check her hot little body from head to toes, look for suspicious rashes on her skin, look for any joints that seem swollen or tender. You better feel the soft spot on the top of her head—if it's bulging, you're going to worry about meningitis, no matter what shots she's had. If it's sunken, you're going to worry that she's dehydrated—maybe she hasn't been drinking well because she feels so rotten, and her body is using more fluid than usual because she's so hot and her metabolism has speeded up. But if you really think there's nothing else wrong, we're going to let you call this a probable viral illness. Maybe you'll decide to check her urine—but you don't have to put her in the hospital for that. Send the urine to the lab, and send the baby home. Spare at least a few seconds' thought for the many connections between what you do as a doctor and all that has been done before you.

When I say all that has been done before you, I don't mean just the technical advances. I also mean the weight of the accumulated and accumulating research. You will be expected to learn to practice medicine with formal reference to all of that research, in a much more systematic way than I did. You are going to train in the era of evidence-based medicine. Evidence-based medicine, or EBM, is the medical profession's attempt to call us to account for our clinical decision making, to ask doctors to stop and think, as they manage patients, whether they are actually applying what is known about that particular condition, that particular medication, that particular procedure. Medicine has its folklore and its pseudoscience as well as its science, and no patient should ever undergo an expensive test or a painful procedure that has been shown not to be effective in that particular clinical setting just because a doctor hopes it might help.

This evidence can be difficult to gather and difficult to analyze. Consider, for example, the story of the Swan-Ganz catheter. When I was a resident, sick and unstable patients in the adult intensive care unit would get a Swan-Ganz catheter. This involved threading a line into one of the large veins in the body, usually the internal jugular in the neck or the subclavian vein under the clavicle, following the blood vessel into the heart, first the right atrium and then the right ventricle, and it allowed the doctors to make important direct measurements. You could monitor the pressure in the lungs, and you could assess the fluid balance of your critically ill patient. When epidemiologists first pointed out that the use of Swan-Ganz catheters was associated with a high death rate, the intensive care specialists were not particularly surprised: The patients in whom these devices were used were the sickest and most unstable patients to start with—that was why there was a high risk of death.

But there was still concern that the monitoring devices, the catheters themselves, might be increasing the risk of death. They had passed into common use in intensive care units without any major studies being done, precisely because they did provide such useful data. The best way to answer the question would have been a randomized trial—manage some of the very sick patients with Swan-Ganz monitoring, and others without it. But intensivists felt so strongly about the value of the catheters that they thought it would be unethical to manage any very sick, very unstable patients in another way. Instead, complex statistical analyses were done, which continued to suggest that the catheters were in fact associated with a higher death rate—and when the randomized study was eventually done, it confirmed the association, and unstable ICU patients are no longer routinely managed with Swan-Ganz catheters. Here were highly trained doctors doing something they believed was clearly helpful from case to case—and in fact, it was increasing the patients' danger. Before you do something to a patient, you have to ask whether it helps, whether it hurts, or whether it does nothing—and you have to ask it in a rigorous scientific way. As you move along your evidence-based way, remember to be humble. The collective wisdom of the smartest doctors in the world doesn't always look so wise in retrospect.

So evidence-based medicine will be a big deal in your training. In the rule-out I previously discussed, for example, my decision in the 1980s to do a sepsis workup on that baby would have been based on a series of studies documenting that the likelihood of a severe bacterial infection increased as you looked at younger children with higher fevers. Your decision in the year 2007 *not* to do a sepsis workup will be based on newer studies, from the era of the new vaccines, that demonstrate the greatly reduced odds of those serious infections.

We do our best to be evidence-based today. There are tools that will be available to you that never existed when I was in school—your ability to search the medical literature from any computer in the hospital, to answer complex medical questions by searching special databases. We've come a long way from the ritual of sending the medical student to the medical library to "pull some papers"—photocopy a few random journal articles and hand them out at attending rounds so that everyone could nod seriously and add them to the moldering pile of photocopied journal articles we all lugged around and stuffed into our backpacks and stacked perilously in the on-call rooms . . . and rarely read, I'm afraid.

In contrast, let's imagine ourselves back in that exam room, with that hot baby. In fact, let's allow you to leave the exam room, with some relief, and ask the nurse to give the baby some ibuprofen. Meanwhile, as you're waiting for the fever to come down, you sit down at one of the computer terminals at the central workstation, and you go to PubMed, a database maintained by the National Library of Medicine and the National Institutes of Health (go ahead, go to www.pubmed.gov—anyone can play). You ask it to search for, oh, let's see, you type in a set of key words, *febrile infant, lumbar puncture, pneumococcal vaccine*. . . . And then you press a search button, and instantly you are looking at the following abstract from the August 2006 issue of *Pediatric Emergency Care*: "Impact of the pneumococcal conjugate vaccine in the management of highly febrile children aged 6 to 24 months in an emergency department." By reading through the abstract, you will learn that few children are getting lumbar punctures and blood cultures today. But you'll still have some questions. Your baby, after all, is not yet fully immunized—she's six months old, so she's had the first three doses of the vaccine, but not the fourth. So you'll keep searching. You'll find some directly relevant studies, and a certain amount of confusion, because no one is going to have done the study of your dreams—a series of children of this exact age and vaccine status. But you'll get to read a 2006 study, "An analysis of pediatric blood cultures in the postpneumococcal conjugate vaccine era in a community hospital emergency department," demonstrating that most blood cultures that did turn positive in this group of children turned out to be false positives—skin organisms that got into the needle and into the blood culture bottles. A number of studies will point you in the direction we discussed; they will reassure you that serious bacterial illness is much less likely than it used to be in the baby you're seeing, but they will still leave the burden of decision on you, according to how sick she looks.

You will train in an era in which you will be expected to justify clinical decision making step by step with medical evidence. You are, like everyone your age, far better at navigating the Internet and finding the specific information you need than I am. If I had asked you to answer the clinical question above and given you no heavy-handed guidance, you might have asked the question more specifically (maybe you would have started with the index of key words, or maybe you already have a patient-management database you really like) and answered it more efficiently.

I also believe that for these same reasons, you will do better at managing the load of incoming medical information and progress than I do. I recently interviewed a residency candidate who told me about an article in the

*New England Journal of Medicine* that had really impressed him. When I said it sounded interesting but I hadn't seen it (after all, it was his job to impress me, not my job to impress him), he offered to send it to me. Sure enough, next day I got a polite e-mail thanking me for the nice interview, with a beautiful PDF of the journal article attached. I was deeply impressed that he could so efficiently retrieve it, attach it, send it—I, who, like so many of my generation, still live with reproachful decades-out-of-date piles of unread medical journals.

Many medical schools and residency programs even teach information management as part of the approach to evidence-based medicine. This really is a field in which you get to keep learning, in which you *must* keep learning. The more systematic you are about figuring out how to manage information, the better. And the more systematic you are about applying that information to clinical questions, the more you'll be doing it right.

I do, however, have to end by warning you that evidence-based medicine is not the whole story. Doctors are human, patients are human; personality and luck and common sense and comfort all play a role in deciding what to do at clinical decision points. One of the pieces you might find in consulting PubMed is a 2006 article from the journal *Pediatrics* titled "The role of parental preferences in the management of fever without source among 3- to 36-month-old children: a decision analysis." This hypothetical study looked at what would happen if, given the risk factors for serious bacterial disease, parents of young children with high fevers were given the choice of whether their children should be treated for possible bacterial infection (your classic rule-out), should be tested but not treated (get the blood culture, get the lumbar puncture, but then send the baby home and leave her alone unless something grows), or should just be observed (tell the parents, take her home and call us if she gets any sicker). The authors concluded that with the vaccine the risks are low with all three strategies, and that it would therefore be reasonable for physicians to take parental preference into account when deciding how to manage any individual child. In other words, it was an evidence-based argument for not having a single evidence-based management approach.

The hospital politics of decision making by groups of different doctors, representing different specialties and different levels of seniority, remain anthropologically complex. Two physicians, David Isaacs and Dominic Fitzgerald, published an article in the distinguished *British Medical Journal* pointing out a variety of alternative decision-making systems. For example, instead of evidence-based medicine, you can practice eminence-based medicine, in which the most prominent doctor at the table gets the final say. Or there's vehemence-based medicine, in which the doctor who speaks most emphatically (read, yells the loudest) makes the call. Or there's eloquence-based medicine, in which the decision is made according to which physician is the best orator, and perhaps the suavest dresser. If all else fails, there's providence-based medicine, in which you leave it up to God. And I should mention that another doctor, Arthur M. Lam, wrote to the journal to suggest the following: "I wish to add arrogance-based medicine to the list, although I recognise that it overlaps with eminence-based medicine and eloquence-based medicine. It is particularly relevant in teaching hospitals, where opinions are given out as fact and no explanations are needed. The measuring device is phrase count; the unit of measurement is the phrase 'because I said so.'"

# 6

## ▩ Against Medical Advice

*The patient is a twenty-five-year-old female, gravida one, para zero to one, who has reached her EDC and gone into early labor. She has had an uneventful pregnancy, has no known drug allergies, and is on no medications, other than prenatal vitamins. She has a deep distrust of medical interventions, and expresses the desire to undergo labor with no IV, with no anesthesia or analgesia, and with no fetal monitoring. She informs the nurses in labor and delivery that she intends to leave the hospital as soon as her baby is delivered.*

*Dear Orlando,*

That was me, your mother the medical student, in labor with you, my first child. That's what gravida one means—pregnant for the first time. Para zero to one means I was going from never having given birth to giving birth for the first time. It's one of those secret medical notations—you'll see it at the beginning of any written medical history of a woman who has reached what we call "reproductive age." It can be a telling little abbreviation; G4P1, for example, means she's been pregnant four times, but only given birth once, so that means three pregnancies ended, either by miscarriage or by therapeutic abortion. That's a lot of life history and medical event packed into two letters and two numbers. The EDC is the due date, but the abbreviation hangs on from the dear dead days when we referred to a woman's labor as her "confinement"—an EDC is an estimated date of confinement, calculated at forty weeks from the beginning of the last menstrual period before pregnancy, or about thirty-eight weeks from conception. Is that more than you want to know about your own gestation?

Anyway, there I was, on my due date, in labor with my first child—with you—and I just hated being a patient. You know what? I still hate it. A few months ago I went into the hospital for day surgery. I had what my doctor thought might be some polyps in my uterus, so they were going to be removed. I hadn't eaten since before midnight the night before, as instructed, and I ended up waiting around for hours because the operating room was backed up. Finally I changed into my johnny (I hate wearing a johnny), and they took away my eyeglasses (I hate giving up my eyeglasses), and they put an IV in my hand (I hate IVs), and they gave me some wonderful, relaxing drug (I did my labors without drugs, but I have to admit I like those sedatives!). I went right to sleep and woke up a little later with the operation successfully completed. Then I drove the nurses in the recovery room crazy—they wanted me to lie quietly for a while, then sit for a while, then sip some ice water, make sure I was steady, and they would call my husband and tell him I'd be ready to go in an hour or so. But there I was, standing up shakily on the tile floor, two minutes after opening my eyes, demanding my eyeglasses, my clothing. My glasses, where have you put my glasses, give me my glasses! Can we please get this IV out of my hand, NOW! They told me to take it easy, I might be woozy, I might fall. But I was pulling on my clothing under the johnnies, throwing the johnnies on the floor, secretly calling your father on my cell phone to tell him to hurry up and come get me. There was this perfectly nice nurse whose sacred responsibility it was to escort me out of the hospital and hand me over to Larry (because, after all, I might faint or fall—I had just woken up, I had just had a surgical procedure), and I practically ran through the halls with the poor woman chugging along in my wake, I was so eager to get away.

Why do I hate being a patient so much? It wouldn't be fair to say that I hate hospitals. I made professional choices that meant spending years of my life working in hospitals, and I like them. When I visit a new hospital—to see a friend, to give a talk—I always walk right in and feel at home. I feel entitled to ride in the "staff only" elevators and find my way through the corridors without worrying that I'm venturing off-limits. There are plenty of people who plain hate hospitals, including many of my close relatives, but I am always surprised by their emotion. My own mother—your grandmother—hates hospitals. They remind her of illness and mortality and fear; they are filled with sick people and with incomprehensible machines; they are inhabited by authority figures in scrubs and nursing uniforms and white coats who must not under any circumstances be questioned or defied but who evoke a certain amount of mistrust and hostility. I am one of those authority figures. When I think about the tests and the procedures that frighten my mother, I think of them mostly in terms of the information they yield. The people who work in the hospital are doing good and necessary work, and odds are, they're reasonably good, reasonably smart people, drawn to work I understand.

But boy, oh boy, do I not want to be their patient! I do not want to be in the power of these reasonably good, reasonably smart people, doing their good and necessary work. Take away my medical identity, make me into a patient, and suddenly I have all my mother's fears and anxieties mixed together with my own doctorly sense of arrogance and entitlement. Don't think I'm going to follow your stupid rules. Get away from me with your dangerous, mind-clouding medications. Let me out of this johnny! Let me out of this room! And I don't think this is either a terrible fear of pain (I'm the one who preferred the pain of childbirth to the medical indignity of an IV to give me painkillers, let alone an epidural catheter to administer true anesthesia) or even a terrible fear of my own mortality. No, I think it's a fear of being a patient, pure and simple, a fear of being powerless in a setting where I expect to feel in control.

During my twenties, I was that standard cliché, the woman who goes to the doctor only when she's pregnant. It was an interesting experience, being pregnant in medical school. I quickly realized I didn't want to think of myself as a patient. I didn't mind the scientific side of it so much, although I admit it was sometimes hard to think about all the ways that embryologic development could go awry. But my defenses were generally good. After all, if I could sit through lecture after lecture on the things that could go wrong with the body—the heart, the lungs, the gastrointestinal system—and not worry that they were going wrong with *my* body, then why shouldn't I feel similarly immune on my fetus's behalf?

Some medical students aren't able to manage that imaginary immunity. In fact, there's that recognized medical student syndrome that I mentioned earlier in which some students—the ones with vivid imaginations—compare their own symptoms with each new interesting syndrome as it's presented in lecture, and diagnose themselves left and right, in some cases examining themselves and finding suspicious (if subtle) physical findings. They're given to checking their own pulses for irregularities that may denote life-threatening arrhythmias, anxiously taking their own blood pressures and finding them (anxiously) elevated.

You'll find medical student syndrome described in Wikipedia; it's a specific form of hypochondria. And you can understand how it works. Any normal person, reading, say, a magazine article about the insidious onset of certain forms of cancer might feel the urge to check for enlarged lymph nodes just along the collar bone (so much more suspicious than lymph nodes in the neck!). Anyone hearing that certain memory slips can presage early-onset Alzheimer's would naturally feel inclined to try to answer the handily supplied test-your-memory questions in the article sidebar, just to show a mind in good working order. When you're a medical student, you hear about these signs and symptoms all day long, learning details about diseases you had never even imagined.

So you can give way to medical student syndrome and diagnose yourself—or sometimes a family member—with each new terrible disease that comes your way, no matter how unlikely. (*Today I learned that colon cancer in its early stages can be without any symptoms—hey, I don't have any symptoms. . . . Oh, no, I must have colon cancer!*) Or you can move psychically in the opposite direction and refuse to consider the possibility that any of the information you're so busy memorizing might apply to you. These are similar reactions—turned inside out—to the influx of new and important and scary information about all the bad things that can happen, and to the pressure to absorb and process and remember that information.

Looking back, I think I regarded pathophysiology too much as a kind of interesting zoological survey: These are the strange and terrible things that can happen to people. Not to me, you understand, but to *people*. It was my defense against the harshest lesson of medical school, which is also the harshest lesson of practicing medicine: that we are all living in vulnerable bodies that are susceptible to illness of all kinds, and that will, inevitably, encounter damage and decay. I suspect that the people who palpate swollen lymph nodes in their own neck regions while studying lymphoma and feel their muscles weakening as they read about multiple sclerosis are, in fact, coming to terms with their own humanity and vulnerability, even as they wander over the line into true, if transient, hypochondria. No, it isn't happening to them, but it could, and that's not a bad thing for a medical student to remember.

But as a pregnant medical student, I had the other reaction to what I studied in pathophysiology: *None of this is happening to me, none of this will ever happen to me.* It's interesting material, yes, and I have to learn it, but for the sake of my patients. Yes, I admit I squirmed a bit during those second-year pathophysiology courses as I learned the details of each and every genetic defect—while all the while there you were, your genetic makeup already determined, growing and developing in utero. Yes, I moaned and groaned a little, for form's sake, about how yucky it was to have to memorize long lists of birth defects while waiting for my own due date. But I think what really bothered me was the idea that when my due date came, I would be transformed inexorably into a patient.

Even way back then I was a grumpy patient. You were born in a teaching hospital. It was a community hospital, because I didn't want to go to one of the big academic hospitals (actually, at the time, we didn't have a car, and you were due in January, in the middle of the New England winter, and I didn't want to risk going into labor and having to find a taxi into Boston—the community hospital was in Cambridge, and in a pinch, I thought, I could walk over). But it was a teaching hospital, and there were medical students around, doing their OB/GYN rotations. I made it absolutely clear that there were to be no medical students allowed anywhere near me when I was in labor. I didn't want to see anyone I might have met—or might one day meet—over at the medical school. I didn't want anyone in the room who was any kind of a beginner.

I'm still a terrible patient, in every sense. I do now have a primary-care physician of my own, and I have gone for a checkup almost every year for the past four or five years. My doctor wants me to eat properly, and she gets a missionary light in her eye when she talks about grilled fish and steamed broccoli. I even believe she herself follows this advice—she speaks like someone who would not ask me to do something she would not do herself—and I do believe she gets up early every morning to exercise and that gives her a jump on the whole day. I wish I did that too—but I don't, and I'm not going to, and I can see she looks at me and thinks I should really know better. After all, I'm a doctor.

But I'm not the only one. I once put the question to a group of doctors who take care of adults as well as children: *Do you follow your own advice? Do you follow your doctor's advice?* Everyone laughed. Absolutely not, said one young doctor, why, I don't even *have* a doctor. And they went around the room with pretty much the same story. I'm too busy to eat properly, I grab junk food. When I'm feeling sick or low-energy, I assume it's because I'm working too hard and not getting enough sleep. I don't want any of the workup that I would do for one of my patients with those complaints—I know there's nothing really wrong with me.

That's probably a big part of it: *I know there's nothing really wrong with me.* Doctors have the ability to create medical denial from our expertise and our experience. Assiduously avoiding medical student syndrome, you separate yourself from the category of "the patient," the person to whom illnesses happen. When your patient feels unusually fatigued, you the doctor worry about anemia, or even maybe about malignancy. When you yourself feel fatigued, there's nothing unusual about it and nothing worth working up. When the patient has an unusually bad headache, you do a careful neurologic exam. When you have one, you know it's just overwork and stress. Diseases are bad things that happen to patients; we are not patients. We are a race apart. And because we are a race apart, we don't always have to follow our own advice, no matter how worthy, no matter how evidence-based.

Giving advice is easy; following advice is hard—for everyone, not just for doctors. During my career as a doctor and a writer, I have made a mild specialty of admitting that I can't always follow my own advice. When you were a baby, Orlando, I admitted—in print!—that I sometimes put you to bed with a bottle. Pediatricians fight an endless battle against bedtime bottles, which are linked to bad tooth decay, ear infections, and heaven knows what else. I conscientiously urge the parents of my patients to do away with that go-to-sleep bottle. So why did I let you drink one, even occasionally? Because it helped you fall asleep, and to help you fall asleep, I would have put you to bed with any damn thing you wanted. I made fun of myself for falling short of being the pediatric parenting paragon I wanted to be.

Many pediatricians who are also parents suffer from this stress. Your child has a meltdown in the toy store over something he feels he cannot live without and you finally begin screaming at him. Then, look, here comes a family you take care of, the children advancing toward you, surprised to see you in this unfamiliar setting, followed by a parent with a quizzical look on her face. *Doctor, was that you I just heard screaming threats of physical violence?* So you hastily hand your child the toy he was screaming for (no doubt a plastic submachine gun with authentic details and particularly loud sound effects) and get the hell out of there, permanently humiliated as a parent, a physician, a parenting expert, and a human being. In a similar spirit, I have an internist friend who was approached by a patient while he was enjoying a steak in a restaurant, and had to listen to a gleeful little speech about cholesterol. See, Doc, you tell me to cut back on the red meat, and look at you!

The ways I fall short of the goals I professionally and glibly recommend to others give me a certain realism, I suppose, and a certain understanding of the challenges of real life. It is possible that our problematic habits make us better advice givers, more respectful of our patients' struggles, more compassionate about their failings. On the other hand, I feel I have become much worse at receiving advice from my doctor, and less respectful of her feelings as a caregiver. I still nod and smile when she talks about exercise, but my expression is obviously somewhat cynical, somewhat dubious, and I occasionally find myself interrupting her good advice to tell her that this or that or the other thing just isn't going to happen. I am *not* going to restructure my life so that I get up an hour earlier and exercise and get a jump on the day. I hate the early morning, and I have always hated the early morning, and I already get up way earlier than I want to, and whatever time I get up, anyway, the whole day and everything I need to do comes crashing into my brain and I start to feel overwhelmed and under pressure—and never mind. I don't want to say all this to my doctor, either, because I'm afraid she'll try to put me on an antidepressant. Instead, I shrug and I say, *well, you may be right, well, I'll try*—I don't believe myself, and I can see she doesn't believe me either, but she's probably tired of me and tired of giving good advice to someone who should know better already, and by mutual discouraged agreement we move on.

You will find that medical training is full of stories about specialists who were so immersed in denial that they were caught off guard by their own diagnoses. When I asked those young doctors if they followed their own medical advice, one of them offered a story about a cardiologist too distinguished to be named who felt some tightness in his chest and wrote it off to muscle strain, until it was almost too late. In other words, he missed his own heart attack. Seasoned doctors too will tell you about the oncologist who never bothered with his own screening colonoscopy, or the infectious diseases expert who ate sushi in some dubious places and picked up a fascinating parasite. These stories—and I would bet that many of them are urban doctor legends—resonate because they offer medical drama, medical irony, and the always-disconcerting reminder that, in fact, we have no professional immunity whatsoever. The things that make other people sick make us sick as well; the risk factors and the warning signs that we advise our patients to heed carefully are also intimations of our own frailty and mortality. Just because you know the human heart inside out—its anatomy and physiology, its electromechanical conduction, its rhythms and arrhythmias—well, all that does not strengthen your own heart muscle one iota.

Speaking of hearts, I recently read a fascinating doctor-as-patient story on the front page of the *New York Times* about Dr. Michael DeBakey, who devised the surgery to repair what are called dissecting aortic aneurysms. An aortic aneurysm is a kind of bubble in the wall of the aorta, the big mother artery that takes oxygenated blood out of the left ventricle and carries it out to reach the rest of the body. If the wall of the aorta is weakened—by years of high blood pressure, or by injury, or by certain genetic conditions—a bubble can develop in between the different layers of the vessel wall. If that bubble starts to spread, with air separating out the layers, you have a dissecting aortic aneurysm. It usually hurts a lot, and it's life-threatening in a major way; if the aorta ruptures because the walls are weakened and thinned out by this dissection process, you die.

Dr. DeBakey developed the surgery to repair these aneurysms—and then, at the age of ninety-seven, he developed one himself. He diagnosed himself, made the decision not to undergo surgery because of his age, and hoped that his aorta would heal. But the disease progressed, he was admitted to the hospital, and the final decision to operate was made by the other surgeons, because the patient himself was unconscious. The surgeons wanted to operate; the anesthesiologists refused, according to Dr. DeBakey's wife, because "the anesthesiologists feared that Dr. DeBakey would die on the operating table and did not want to become known as the doctors who killed him." So an anesthesiologist from another hospital, a friend of DeBakey's, was called in for the operation. Meanwhile, the hospital ethics committee held a dramatic last-minute meeting, which was interrupted by the patient's wife, who demanded immediate surgery. There was a seven-hour operation, following Dr. DeBakey's own process, that repaired his aorta, and a long and difficult recovery and rehabilitation. A year later, at the time of the news story, he was "back working nearly a full day."

There you have a doctor who found himself a patient, being treated, in a sense, by doctors who were advised by his own shadow. You have a doctor who made the rules and broke the rules, you have a doctor making his own diagnosis and attempting to manage his own care, you have colleagues who feel a special loyalty, but also maybe colleagues who feel a special anxiety about treating a star in their profession. This one story covers just about every possible permutation of the doctor trying to be his own doctor, as well as the doctor being cared for by other doctors.

A friend of mine, an internist, successfully diagnosed his own appendicitis. It's another great doctor-as-patient story, and here's how it happened. He went to bed one night with a queasy stomach and thought he must have eaten something that disagreed with him. The next morning he still felt queasy, so he figured he must have some kind of stomach flu because it was lasting too long to be food-related. He did what any sensible doctor would do who found himself feeling sick with something probably contagious: he went to work and saw patients (*how can I justify staying home from work just because I don't feel well, that would be wimpy, I'm not so sick as all that—not like a patient*). However, by the time he was in clinic, he noticed that the pain had localized to the right lower quadrant of his abdomen—and he knew (as even many non-physicians know) that lower right-sided pain is the absolute hallmark of appendicitis. Still, he was inclined to dismiss this (*of course I don't have appendicitis, don't be ridiculous, how could I have appendicitis*). He did take the trouble to examine himself, and he noticed that when he pressed hard on his lower right abdomen it hurt a little, but if he then took his hand away quickly it hurt much more (*well, that certainly seems like a classic rebound tenderness sign, the kind you're taught to look for with appendicitis, and I'm not sure I've ever elicited it so clearly in one of my patients—but that doesn't mean I have appendicitis, no sir, not me!*). So he started to walk home, but he couldn't make it because it hurt too much to put pressure on his right foot.

Finally he turned back toward the hospital and walked (hobbled) into the emergency room, introduced himself to the attending doctor, and said he had appendicitis. Let him tell the story: "I said, 'I have appendicitis.' She said, 'Really?' I said, 'Yes, I have appendicitis.' She put me in a room and the surgeon came in and said, 'Yes, you have appendicitis.' So they took out my appendix. Of course, I wanted to stay in the hospital for as little time as possible, so the next morning when the surgeon came for the 4 a.m. rounds, I said, 'What do I have to do to leave?' He said that usually people leave after two or three days. So I said, 'I know that, but what do I have to do to leave?' He said, 'You have to be able to eat and walk around.' I ate my breakfast, and it didn't come up. Then I walked around the ward. I got back into bed, called the nurse, and told her I wanted to leave the hospital. She looked at me dubiously and said she would call the resident. After a long time, she got the resident, a first-year surgical intern. I told the intern I was ready to leave, and he said that wasn't possible. I said, 'Yes, it's possible. You just need to tell your chief resident I'm ready to go.' He left the room looking extremely frightened, and he never came back."

I listen to this story and I think about that poor surgical intern, who probably believed that if he let this patient leave, the morning after his appendectomy, the patient might go home and die, and it would be his, the intern's, fault. Or maybe he was terrified of calling the surgical chief resident; surgical chief residents are powerful, and interns aren't supposed to bother them about silly details. You call the chief if someone's bleeding to death, or if someone's heart stops beating. But maybe he sucked it up and called the chief, and the chief said, I'm in the operating room, saving lives, and you come bothering me with this crap. Go back and talk to the patient and explain why he needs to stay for his own safety. Or maybe he put off calling the chief because he was scared, or maybe he got paged about four other patients and got busy doing some other piece of intern scut.

My friend continues his story.

"So when no chief resident came, I called the head of the hospital, and said, 'You need to get the surgical attending to come discharge me, or else I am going to sign out AMA, and that looks very bad for your hospital.' So she got the attending out of a meeting, and he came and signed me out; he made it clear that this was not the usual practice, but he was willing to do it."

Let me tell you about signing out against medical advice (AMA). That's the locution doctors use when we want to document that we did our best to prevent a patient from taking a risk, and the patient refused to listen. Usually it refers to leaving the hospital or the emergency room when the doctor thinks the patient may be unstable. You tell someone that in your best judgment he needs a spinal tap—or an emergency cardiac catheterization, or an ICU admission—and the patient says, no way I'm doing that, I'm out of here! Or you try to explain to the patient why it's important to stay for a few more days of antibiotic treatment, or why his blood pressure is dangerously out of control, and he says, forget it, I feel fine! Then you document that in the chart. Finally, you always ask patients to sign a special form acknowledging that you are advising them not to leave for their own good.

Whenever you have to document one of those AMA results, you feel you've failed. You didn't really explain things to the patient properly, you didn't communicate the risk, you didn't reassure a frightened patient. Somehow, the doctor-patient relationship went wrong, and the patient is at risk. So the idea of a sensible, senior academic internist threatening to sign out AMA is a little peculiar.

"Great work," I said to him. "You are a true paradigm of the physician-patient. I'm sure they're still telling the story. Anything else you'd like to say?"

He thought for a minute. "Well," he said, "I didn't go to my post-op visit because I knew there was no reason to."

I understood perfectly, and I identified with his story completely, because I went through a version of the same thing back when you were born, Orlando. It turned out to be a long and difficult labor, more than twenty-four hours. When you finally put in an appearance, I was exhausted. I didn't forget that my plan had been for early discharge—they were supposed to let me go home four hours after the delivery. But because the labor was so long and the doctor had gotten anxious, he suggested that I stay overnight and rest, stay and let them monitor me. I have only the haziest recollection of this whole interaction, but your father swears that the next thing he knew I was sitting up in bed clutching you and demanding to know why I had to stay. "What are you worried about, my blood pressure?" he remembers me saying. "There wasn't much blood loss, was there?"

They did let me go—let us go—four hours later, and we were fine. For that matter, my friend did go home the day after his appendectomy, and he was fine too. I guess it's generally true that medicine attracts people who like to be in charge and relish the decision maker's role. Our training leaves us feeling as if we're especially entitled to that role in anything that has to do with health. Lots of doctors do take care to follow their own advice, and all of us try to follow at least some of it. When I don't, I feel guilty about it—a strong sense of foolish I-should-know-better-than-this-but-I-don't, a generalized hostility that I should properly direct at myself but that manifests itself in a kind of irritation at my doctor. It's almost as if I expect her to let down her guard and admit that all this advice is strictly a theoretical construct—we don't really expect anyone to listen to us, do we?

Maybe I was better once about believing that I really would follow her advice; maybe I believed more whole-heartedly that I might turn over a new leaf once and for all. Maybe it's really now in my overweight, disagreeable middle age that I have come to respond to good advice about diet and exercise with a cynical shrug—cynical not about the value of the advice but about my own ability to follow it. I have lost—to my regret—some big part of my self-deception, and along with it, I have lost some part of my willingness to deceive others in the name of kind-ness, or even professional solidarity. On the other hand, I have gained a hard-won understanding about the diffi-culty of turning over those new leaves, a respect for the struggle and dedication that keep people turning them over, bit by bit, and admiration for the doctors who find ways to help them do it.

Orlando, a little human frailty makes us better doc-tors, makes us more able to imagine, understand, and occasionally even alleviate the struggles our patients en-dure. You may not want to admit it any more than I did, but, in fact, we are all patients, all of us. All our lives. We have no immunity—not against the various diseases we study, not against bad habits and lapses of judgment, not against dumb decisions, and not against bad luck. You should use that knowledge—even the scary and frustrating aspects of it—as you turn into a physician.

As your mother, I hope that you do take proper care of your health, that you don't ignore it when your body is telling you something's wrong, that you get proper medical care and watch what you eat, and that you don't ever find yourself using alcohol or tobacco or any kind of drug or even food to take the pain out of a difficult existence. Recognize your vulnerability and use it to understand your patients, but at the same time, take good care of yourself. Don't kid yourself that you're in some other category of humanity, walled safely off from all the consequences of stress, cholesterol, or hereditary disease. Because you'll be a doctor, but you'll also be a patient—as are we all.

## 7

## ▨ Making Mistakes

*A twenty-four-year-old man presents to your clinic with headache, nasal discharge, and low-grade fevers. His paper chart is not available, but he tells you he is homeless and has been living on the street, but that he is basically healthy except for some stomach problems for which he sometimes takes pills that another doctor at the clinic has given him. On physical exam, he is tired-appearing, with dark circles below both eyes. He is not in any respiratory distress. He has some sinus tenderness and bilateral cervical lymph node swelling; his throat exam is normal. His lung fields are clear bilaterally, and his cardiac exam is normal. You diagnose sinusitis and prescribe antibiotics. Your patient, who is clearly familiar with the clinic, asks if you have any samples you can give him, since he is without medical insurance, and when you look in the sample closet, you do indeed find some samples of a new high-powered antibiotic, which you give him. About two hours later his chart appears on your desk and as you page through it you discover that the stomach medication he is taking is actually a new antireflux drug with which you are not completely familiar—presumably because those were the samples available at that visit. Dutifully, you look up the drug, only to discover that it should under no circumstances be combined with the antibiotic you gave the patient, because together they can cause fatal cardiac arrhythmias. You have no way of contacting the patient; you call the local homeless shelter, but they have never heard of him.*

*Dear Orlando,*

Welcome to the wonderful world of medical error. I could give you so many examples, some of them hypothetical, some of them there-but-for-the-grace-of-God, some of them the ones I made myself. As a medical student on the hospital wards, you will go in terror of making a mistake and hurting a patient—at least, you will go in terror if you have any sense. You won't know much, and you'll be around very sick people. In a good program no one is going to give you enough responsibility to let you be much of a risk. If they aren't watching you carefully, the people supervising you are the ones who aren't living up to their responsibilities. But medical training is structured so that you always feel out there at the limits of your competence, you always feel insecure, you always feel you might make a mistake. As a resident, you will worry about this all the time, and again, your worrying will show that you are essentially in touch with reality. You will have a tremendous amount of responsibility and you'll be working hard and the decisions you make—good or bad—will affect people's lives. Go ahead, worry.

The worry doesn't go away when you finish your training. Every doctor worries about making mistakes, and the intensity doesn't necessarily diminish as you get older and more experienced. Some of the worries are specific to particular fields of medicine. I once gave a talk to an audience of psychiatrists, in which I discussed my middle-of-the-night pediatrician anxieties about having made a poor judgment call or a bad decision. I spoke about lying awake and worrying that a child somewhere was getting sicker or even dying because I had failed to recognize meningitis, or failed to appreciate the intensity of an asthma attack, or had written the wrong prescription. During the question-and-answer period, one of the psychiatrists got up to assure me that unless I had taken care of a large number of seriously suicidal patients, and had lain awake worrying about whether I had assessed them properly, I had never known true middle-of-the-night anxiety. He may have had a point.

Medical errors occur at different levels—the kind you make, the kind you avoid by the skin of your teeth, the kind that somehow get made by the system. Let's talk about how doctors deal with errors, how we deal with the fear of making errors, and how we deal with the knowledge that we've made them. Finally, let's talk about what we are learning about mistakes in hospitals and how often they happen and how you can—at least sometimes—build systems to prevent them.

Let's start with the clinical case above, because it offers us an opportunity to dissect out many different aspects of medical error. There's no question that an error has been made. There's a poor guy out there somewhere on two different medications that are not supposed to be prescribed together, and if he's unlucky the combination might make his heart stop beating—all because he went to see a doctor about his drippy nose and his headaches. Not good.

The first thing we see when we examine this case is that it starts with *good intentions*. You were seeing a homeless patient who had no insurance in a clinic that was presumably set up to deliver good medical care to people in that situation. You took time with him and examined him carefully and made the best diagnosis you could. When he asked you as a favor to give him antibiotic samples he couldn't afford, you came through for him.

Next, let's consider the *systemic problems* that contributed to your mistake. The patient couldn't remember the name of the other medication he was taking, and you couldn't check it because his chart had not yet been found (or, if your clinic had already made the switch to electronic medical records, we could say the system was down for a couple of hours).

However, we also have to take into account your own *ignorance*, or at least the limitations of your knowledge. You probably know a great deal about a great many different drugs, but you don't know everything, and you didn't know enough to look at the antibiotic and think, hmm, aren't there some serious interactions with some different stomach medications? In fact, while you're beating yourself up (and I promise you, you are indeed beating yourself up over this), let's go ahead and call it something beyond ignorance—let's call it *carelessness*. You knew you were prescribing for a patient who was already taking another medication, but did you stop and think it through? Are you sure you didn't just dismiss it? *The guy doesn't even know what he's taking. Who knows if he's actually taking anything at all?* Are you sure you weren't a little more casual about this because he was, in fact, an uninsured homeless person? Can we fix your mistake? Not if we can't find your patient. Maybe there's another little subsidiary mistake here—you should have tried harder to get contact information for your patient. Or you should have had him make a follow-up appointment. If you knew he was slated to come back and be checked in two days, you could at least plan to change the medication.

What would we have to change to prevent your mistake? We could do away with the sample room and the practice of giving out drug samples, which many clinics and hospitals have done for medicolegal reasons. The drug companies are happy to give out samples, hoping that doctors will become more familiar with their products and will start patients on those particular drugs just because the starter doses are available. The medical profession and the hospital licensing authorities worry that that is not the right way to be deciding who should take what medication. In this case they're right, in a certain sense. You chose the antibiotic not after careful thought about the probable causative organisms of sinusitis in a twenty-four-year-old man, and not after giving serious consideration to cost, dosing schedule, palatability, side effects, or, heaven knows, drug interactions. You chose it because when you opened the cabinet, there it was. We could eliminate the cabinet, which would probably make the patient less happy with the clinic, but it would eliminate this particular error.

Or would it? Couldn't you have written the guy a prescription for that exact drug, still without reading his chart, still without figuring out the interaction, still without having any contact information for him? To eliminate this error, maybe we have to fix the system the clinic uses for keeping medical records, either by getting those paper charts up to you more promptly or by fixing those computer glitches.

Wait a minute, though. Even if you'd had the chart in the middle of your busy session, are you sure you would have taken the time to check what other drugs he was taking? Or the time to read up on these medications and their possible interactions? Does it really, in the end, come down to this: that the only way to prevent this medical error is by having smarter, more conscientious doctors?

Of course not, though smarter doctors are always good. But we could build a system to prevent your error if we fixed the computers and if we used, for example, a good electronic medical record system that automatically checked for drug interactions. In other words, when you entered the drug on the patient's medication list, the computer would check the drug you had chosen against all the other drugs on the patient's medication list, and warn you that there was a possible incompatibility. Whew.

Wait another minute. Turns out your colleague didn't enter the stomach drug on the med list. He mentioned it in his note, but since he was just grabbing it out of the med closet, he didn't take the time to open another screen—the medications list screen—and type it in again there. Even if he had, you didn't enter the name of the antibiotic you gave out until much later in the evening, when you were finally typing up your notes. So the information was there in the computer, but it never got to you. True, if both of you had used the computer to generate printed prescriptions, that would have automatically triggered the incompatibility screen, but you didn't do that either.

In order to prevent your error, then, here's what we need to do: Get the clinic to use an appropriate and well-constructed electronic medical record program, without too many clicks or obstacles, train the doctors to use it properly and promptly, and do away with the drug samples. Along the way, we'd like to push for smarter doctors.

We could also turn the question around and ask what the patient could have done to keep himself safe from error. He could have known the name of his own medicine, you might mutter, slightly angry, or he could have maintained a primary-care relationship with a single doctor that would probably have meant better care for him all along. (Treacherously, you may find yourself thinking accusingly that he could have a better living situation and a fixed address where he could be reached and health insurance that would pay for his medications. Before you know it, you're blaming him for everything that's wrong with his life!) The patients who get the best care and are least likely to be hurt by mistakes are the patients who take some responsibility for their own care. They know their medications, even research their medications, and remind their doctors about their problems and their histories. They also question medical decisions and speak up when something seems askew. In other words, they are the privileged, the educated, the empowered, and the self-confident. Your patient certainly doesn't fit the profile.

The good news is that you probably haven't killed your patient. In the end, it's a rare drug interaction, and for all you know he isn't really taking the stomach medicine anymore. You better keep on worrying, though, because if it does kill him, if an ambulance brings him into the emergency room tomorrow and he's pulseless, there is no way you can explain what happened to him without calling it a mistake. Your mistake.

I have made plenty of mistakes like this one. In fact, I based the vignette on a mother who told me clearly that her baby was taking a medication to reduce acid reflux. I nodded and made a note, and then I didn't really think about it as I prescribed an antibiotic for the baby's ear infection. I happily offered the mother a handful of samples, thinking that was pretty helpful of me. Later, after she had gone, I discovered that the two drugs, taken together, could cause fatal arrhythmias. I couldn't reach the mother right away—there was a phone number in the chart, but it turned out to be disconnected, and I had to track her down through the emergency contact number, and so on, and so on. I eventually did track her down, and I told her not to give the baby any of the antibiotic samples, I would call in a prescription for something else. Trust me, I have made plenty of mistakes like this one.

Medical mistakes have been big news lately. In 1999 the Institute of Medicine, which is part of the National

Academy of Sciences, issued a report called "To Err Is Human: Building a Safer Health System," which caused quite a stir—and rightly so. Here's how the report begins:

> *Health care in the United States is not as safe as it should be—and can be. At least 44,000 people, and perhaps as many as 98,000 people, die in hospitals each year as a result of medical errors that could have been prevented, according to estimates from two major studies. Even using the lower estimate, preventable medical errors in hospitals exceed attributable deaths to such feared threats as motor-vehicle wrecks, breast cancer, and AIDS.*

The report went on to sort out the different kinds of errors: diagnostic errors or delays, failure to act on test results, treatment errors and delays, communication errors. This report caused a great deal of debate within the medical profession, a great deal of self-criticism, and a great deal of change—or at least, attempted change. There were researchers who questioned the methods by which those terrifying numbers were arrived at. There was plenty of shame and plenty of accusation. But the report itself tried hard not to point blame. Most medical errors, it said, "do not result from individual reckless-ness. . . . This is not a 'bad apple' problem. More commonly, errors are caused by faulty systems, processes, and conditions that lead people to make mistakes or fail to prevent them."

In other words, when a mistake is made, we need to figure out what in the system allowed it to happen, and rather than blaming the person who made it, we need to figure out how to build some kind of safeguard into the system. There are currently many initiatives under way to do just that. They aren't all new. If you have surgery, all kinds of precautions are in place—some of them as basic as writing on your skin with Magic Marker to be sure no one operates on the wrong side of your body. You would probably understand that they are writing on your body with Magic Marker because sometime, somewhere, some doctor removed the wrong kidney, or the wrong breast. If you have ever had a blood transfusion, you've seen the drill in which nurses check and double-check and triple-check your identity and your blood type and the name on the blood that's come from the blood bank—again because mistakes have been made, and transfusing the wrong blood into a patient is a terrible, often fatal, mistake.

After the Institute of Medicine report, the U.S. government got involved, with congressional hearings on how to keep patients safe, and with a new watchdog group, the Agency for Healthcare Research and Quality. The news media were all over the IOM report, publishing appropriately terrifying articles about whether going to the hospital was terribly dangerous. More recently, in 2006, the IOM published another report specifically addressing the issue of medication errors: giving the wrong drug or the wrong dose or giving it wrong (giving something too quickly through an IV, or wrongly mixed), confusing two similarly named drugs, giving incompatible drugs. The report estimated that 1.5 million Americans are harmed—made sick, injured, or killed outright—every year by medication errors.

In response to reports like these, the medical profession is trying hard to study itself. You can find journal articles now on any subtopic of medical error. "Systematic review of medication errors in pediatric patients," from the *Annals of Pharmacotherapy 2006*, will remind you that "pediatrics poses a unique set of risks, predominantly because of wide variations in body mass, which requires doses to be calculated individually based on patient age, weight, or body surface area. . . . This increases the likelihood of errors, particularly dosing errors." I am certainly familiar with those. Many medications are dosed by the patient's weight, which means that in pediatrics you would give a fifteen-year-old football player who weighs eighty kilograms (176 pounds) ten times the dose you would give a baby who weights eight. Easy to make mistakes, easy to get a decimal point in the wrong place. Or you could look at "Patterns of errors contributing to trauma mortality: lessons learned from 2,594 deaths," from the *2006 Annals of Surgery*: "Trauma care creates a perfect storm for medical errors: unstable patients, incomplete histories, time-critical decisions, concurrent tasks, involvement of many disciplines, and often junior personnel working after-hours in busy emergency departments." That article covers such mistakes as intubating the patient in the wrong place—putting the breathing tube into the esophagus instead of the trachea—or failing to check for internal bleeding.

Orlando, I guarantee you will feel the reverberations of these controversies and this professional self-examination as you go through your training. When I was training, medical errors were barely discussed. No, that's not fair—they were discussed and worried over endlessly, they shadowed us wherever we went, but we thought of them as individual faults and slips and acts of carelessness. If there were two similar-sounding drugs on the formulary, and the intern gave a verbal order for one and the nurse misheard it and gave another, then that was the nurse's fault for not questioning an unlikely drug choice, or the intern's fault for not verifying the order. Take the code cart, the rolling metal container with all the medications you need for resuscitation, which sits on every hospital ward, ready to be rolled into the room if someone stops breathing or goes into cardiac arrest. If there were two different concentrations of epinephrine on the code cart (there were), and you gave a dose of the wrong concentration in the middle of the high drama of a code, then you should beat

yourself up over it. We knew that nurses sometimes practiced specific error-reduction strategies, verifying doses of
drugs, going through an elaborate sponge-counting drill
at the end of surgical procedures to make sure nothing
was inadvertently left inside a patient. But by and large as
fledgling doctors, we were left to make up our own
mistake-avoidance strategies. So you would carry a
crumpled code card listing the correct doses of all those
resuscitation medications in the pocket of your scrubs to
check even the most basic doses when it came down to
life or death. You would invent mnemonics or rules of
memory or eagerly copy them down when other people
suggested them, because otherwise you might forget
some vitally important thing just when it counted most.
The most basic mnemonic is the ABC's—check airway
before you check breathing, then check cardiac function—and I'm sure there is many an intern out there
who has run to a code muttering over and over, A-B-C!
Or that basic rule, no pee, no K, which means you can't
add potassium to a patient's IV until you've verified renal
function by seeing that the patient makes urine.

In your training, I hope, you will encounter more systemic solutions. For example, you can build in verifica-
tion systems, with computers and with humans. A
computer can be programmed with the weight of each
pediatric patient and can question your orders if you
seem to be giving too much or too little of a drug. A good
computer program can check for drug incompatibilities,

or even warn you if you are giving a drug that is metabolized in the liver to a patient whose liver isn't working properly. You can build in checks and balances for your personnel as well—set protocols—or even post them, hanging them up in trauma rooms, for example. You can train everyone involved—doctors, nurses, EMTs—to remember a specific drill for checking the placement of a breathing tube (listen for breath sounds, check an x-ray) and make sure everyone knows there is no penalty for reminding the doctor in charge to follow that protocol. None of these changes will necessarily come easily, and none of these changes will eliminate error. But there is a real, concerted attempt under way to change the way the problem is framed, to stop thinking of medical error as simple, careless mistake making, which leads to a sense of shame and to secrecy and cover-ups—and, of course, to lots of TV medical dramas.

What about the other kind of medical error, the error of judgment, the error of missing an important diagnosis? When I can't sleep at night after an evening seeing patients, I frequently suffer from the conviction that I have missed an important diagnosis, or sent home a child who is too sick to be at home. Remember the sepsis workup we did on that feverish six-month-old? During flu season if I work an evening shift in a busy clinic, I might see ten kids with fever. I will go home and worry about the sicker ones. Flu and flu-like viral illnesses can make children miserable with high fevers, aches and pains, wrenching coughs, and shaking chills. What am I at home worrying about? Did that eight-year-old girl really have bacterial pneumonia? Should I have gotten a chest x-ray? I didn't hear any crackles in her lungs, but that was one hell of a nasty cough, and her fever was high. Is she home now fighting to breathe? Is it possible that teenage boy really had meningitis? He said his neck hurt, and I decided it was because of his sore throat, and his strep test was negative, so I told him it was just a virus, but he sure looked sick. Is he home, right now, dying? And what *about* that six-month-old with the temp of 105? I think we were way too cavalier with her just because she was immunized; she should be in the hospital, under observation, getting antibiotics.

Here's the question, though: If one of those fears actually came true, would that be a medical mistake? I looked at each of those patients, I thought about each of those diagnoses, and I made my decision, there in the exam room. What I was doing at home on the couch in the wee hours of the morning was second-guessing myself, doubting my clinical judgment. Is that the same as a medical mistake? There's no question that if I sent a child home with a diagnosis of flu and he had died of meningitis by morning, I would feel I had made a terrible mistake. I would have "missed a meningitis," as we say in pediatrics. I would have harmed a child, or failed to avert harm.

What I want you to see is that the knowledge of having done harm, or having failed to avert it, would hit hard at my entire sense of who I am and what I do. You go into medicine to help and protect and cure. You learn the basic medical injunction, "First, do no harm," in medical school, and you hear it over and over. (You also learn it in Latin, *primum non nocere*, which gives it a certain air of antiquity, though in fact it doesn't seem to date to classical times, and it has nothing to do with the Hippocratic oath, which, in any case, is translated from the Greek.) You are not supposed to hurt people, and when you feel that you have hurt someone, you crumple up.

Beyond the worry, I know that if I see enough patients with high fever during enough clinic sessions, sooner or later one of them is going to have a bad outcome. No matter how carefully I look at each child, no matter how deliberately I make each judgment call, they're still a series of judgment calls, and eventually I'll get one wrong. I'll see a kid who just doesn't look all that sick, but who really has something bad. Or I'll see a kid who has the symptoms of one thing in my examining room, but then goes on to develop something else. Or I'll waver on the border of a decision to send a child to the emergency room and decide, no, he can go home safely. In each of these cases I might call it wrong. That is another major and unresolvable truth of medicine: that bad things happen and there are bad outcomes, and when they happen to your patients, you blame yourself, you feel at fault, and all you can think about is how you could have prevented them. If I ever send a child home and something happens to that child, my judgment will seem to me completely indefensible. How could I not have seen what was coming, how could I have made the wrong call?

There are some fields in which the parameters define a certain rate of bad outcomes. Obstetricians go into the delivery room knowing that some births go wrong, that some babies die at delivery. Surgeons have to operate with the knowledge that some patients don't survive. That's why the malpractice rates are so high for obstetricians and for surgeons—because any delivery or any operation that ends badly may be viewed as the doctor's mistake, and because the question of whether there is in fact any fault involved may well have to be fought out in court.

Am I telling you that there is no such thing as malpractice? Of course not. I have been beating you over the head with the idea that medical practice is full of errors, and that hospitals are dangerous places. There are plenty of operations—or deliveries—where you can make a good case that things weren't done right, or mistakes were made. My father suffered through a badly done GI operation that left him in discomfort for years. Eventually another surgeon had to redo it, and he came about as close as one surgeon will to saying that another hadn't done a proper job. In pediatrics, I heard through the mother grapevine—as opposed to the doctor grapevine—about a parent who repeatedly told the doctor there was something wrong with the way her child was walking, and the doctor shrugged it off. The child turned out to have developmental dysplasia of the hip and needed extensive surgery to correct what could have been fixed much more easily if only the doctor had listened to the mother's original concern. Sometimes people don't practice up to standard, and sometimes certain people are below standard over and over. It happens. But even when you aren't one of those doctors, and you don't make those mistakes, there are going to be a certain number of medical cases that don't go the way we all—doctor and patient and family and hospital—want them to. You as the physician are going to live your professional life dealing with those outcomes, judging yourself, and perhaps being judged. It comes with the territory.

What do we do when we make a mistake, or when we see a mistake get made? In spite of everything I've been saying about the movement to reduce medical error, I think you'll find there's still a tremendous sense of shame, a tendency to blame yourself, not the system—and also still a strong urge to keep errors secret, if they can possibly be kept secret. We have a long way to go if medicine is going to move further toward full disclosure and even apology. Part of this lag is due to the fear of being sued. There has not been any provision at all in medical culture for admitting error, apologizing to injured patients, and making restitution. Instead, the teaching was explicit: If a mistake is made, be careful what you document in the chart, be careful what you say, turn it over to the lawyers, if necessary, but don't make yourself the fall guy. The penalty for being honest could be wildly disproportionate jury awards, could even be your whole career.

There are people who are trying to change this. In particular, there is a relatively new movement to establish a protocol for civilized handling of medical errors: acknowledge the error honestly, apologize to the patient (and mean it!), and build a system in which the hospital offers restitution without waiting to be sued. This may sound obvious to you, or it may sound almost unbelievable—either insane or utopian. Dr. Lucian Leape, a prominent professor of health policy at Harvard who was closely involved with the Institute of Medicine report on medical error, is also involved in the search for nonpunitive ways to deal with errors and is a strong advocate for apology:

> *Full disclosure is the right thing to do. It is not an option; it is an ethical imperative. . . . The case for apology is very different. . . . Apology is not an ethical right, but a therapeutic necessity. Apology makes it possible for the patient to recognize our humanity, our fallibility, our remorse at having caused harm. . . . Apology is necessary for healing, for "getting over it."*

*It doesn't always work. Sometimes the patient's anger is too great for forgiveness. But healing cannot occur without it. To be effective, it must be a true apology, in which the caregiver takes responsibility for the event and shows remorse and a desire to make amends.*

Apologizing is another thing no one ever taught me to do—or even discussed with me—in medical school or in residency. I'll be curious to see whether apologizing figures in your medical education, whether they discuss its place in medical practice and even offer you models. Apologizing is a big change in medical thinking and in medical culture, and if it does become accepted, it's going to take a while. Your generation of doctors is probably going to have to teach mine how to do it.

As a doctor you may find yourself apologizing for a mistake that has caused great pain and suffering, or apologizing to a son or daughter for an error that ended a parent's life. There's no reason the patient—or the patient's family—should necessarily find the apology comforting, or sufficient. I read about one terrible case in a Canadian hospital in which an eleven-year-old girl died after surgery, and the hospital investigated the death and found that the resident had not responded in a timely way to reports that she was having difficulty. The hospital apologized to the parents, acknowledging that different actions might have meant a different outcome—a living child instead of a dead child. The father, who continued to pursue legal action, was in no way satisfied. "There's an issue of personal accountability and responsibility in this death, i.e., physicians," he said. "I use the analogy of the drunk driver killing your child with his car and having the insurance company apologize to you—there's really no gratification in it. Personal accountability and responsibility is nowhere in the system."

Doctors have a lot to learn about how to apologize, and there will always be certain medical situations in which an apology doesn't help. But let me leave you with a few thoughts about error, honesty, and taking care of patients.

Orlando, this is a serious job with serious stakes— life-and-death stakes. You owe the job a conscientious attempt to do it well, to look for possible sources of error and danger and do away with them, even at the cost of significant extra effort. But you need to begin your life in this job with a much less naïve approach to error than I had when I trained. I thought of error as individual, as completely separate from the systems in which I worked, and I thought of it as shameful. If something went wrong, you blamed yourself, you doubted yourself, maybe doubted your whole life, but you kept it to yourself. You didn't write about it in the chart, or discuss it with the patient or the patient's family. You told yourself that error was rare. You told yourself that if you admitted any doubts, you might be set upon by ravening malpractice lawyers who would twist your honesty into ropes and hang you and everyone who worked with you.

I hope you will study and practice in a different environment. I hope you can acknowledge that medical errors are common, and that many of them are closely related to the way we construct our medical systems. I hope your generation of doctors will be more aware of the dangers and more attuned to how to fix them so hospitals become safer for everyone. I hope you will practice in a medical world—and a medicolegal world—that is able to confront more honestly the difficult realities that medicine is not always a certain science, and that bad outcomes occur even with good practice. And I hope that as you train we will make real progress in handling errors and bad outcomes when they do occur so you and your contemporaries will be able to face those life-and-death stakes with greater honesty and with greater understanding.

# 8

## ■ Knowing Stories and Keeping Secrets

*Jeanette, a seventeen-year-old female in good health, presents for her annual physical examination. She is a junior in high school and plans to go on to community college and eventually to become a teacher. She will be the first person in her family to attend college, and in fact the first person in her family to graduate from high school. She has had asthma in the past, but it has not bothered her in several years, though she uses her inhaler occasionally when she has an upper respiratory infection. She denies any cigarette smoking ("it would just make me wheeze"), any alcohol use ("I've seen how that can mess up your life!"), or any drug use ("I stay away from all those people, they are just plain bad news!"). She has a boyfriend but has not been sexually active. On physical exam, her lungs are clear, with no*

*wheezing, and the remainder of her exam is*
*completely normal. As Jeanette is getting dressed*
*to leave, she asks you the following question:*
*"Doctor, how are you supposed to decide about—*
*you know?" You take a guess and say, "Do you*
*mean about having sex with your boyfriend?"*
*Jeanette nods. "Doctor, what do you do when*
*your body really wants to do something, and your*
*brain isn't sure?"*

*Dear Orlando,*

I had taken care of Jeanette since she was five years
old. I knew her whole family. They didn't live in easy circumstances, and she hadn't had an easy life—not much
money, no father in the home. When she was thirteen
years old, and full of anger and rebellion, her mother had
been terrified that Jeanette was running with a bad crowd,
that she was growing up too fast, that she would get pregnant and drop out of school the way people around her
were doing. In fact, her mother had asked me whether I
would be willing to give her shots of Depo-Provera (a
contraceptive) without telling her what I was doing. No, I
had said, I don't think I could do that. I was willing to talk
to her about contraception, I told her mother. But her
mother didn't want me to. "She's too young for that," she
said. It wasn't logical, but you know mothers. . . . So,
Jeanette and I had been around the block together. Every
time I saw her this last year or two, I was stunned by how

confident she was, how lovely she was, how successful she was. She had stayed in school, against what I would once have considered mighty odds, she had done well, and she was graduating and going on to college.

Orlando, you are in people's *lives* when you do this job. I looked at this seventeen-year-old, this beautiful and confident and uncertain and successful and tentative girl, and I was looking at someone whose life had over-lapped with mine for more than a decade. I remember her as a scrappy kid with asthma attacks and patches of eczema on her arms and legs. I remember her as that troubled thirteen-year-old who certainly wasn't going to ask any questions, since she already felt she knew every-thing. I was thinking of rashes and wheezes and school physicals—and a child growing up. I know what you're thinking: In some ways it was like looking at you and thinking of all the children you've been, from that med-ical school baby to that internship toddler to the young man you are today. Except it also wasn't. Sure, there's probably something maternal in the way a pediatrician feels toward her patients, but that's only a small part of the mix. Among other things, I knew my patient was specifically asking me the question she wouldn't ask her mother, and she trusted me to listen and react and an-swer in a way that her mother might not. It's that com-plicated mix of affection and professional investment and academic interest and yes, even detachment, that will shape your life.

"What a good question," I said. I mean, isn't it? What *do* you do when your body really wants to do something and your brain isn't sure? Personally, in that situation, I have a spotty record—sometimes I listen to my brain, and sometimes I don't. So I asked Jeanette to tell me *why* she thought her brain wasn't sure. Was she unsure about the boyfriend or his feelings for her, or hers for him? Did she feel she wasn't ready for the relationship to get more serious? Was he pressuring her? I delivered the little lecture on female sexual pleasure that my colleagues and I always try to give teenage girls in this situation: You are entitled to enjoy what you do sexually (but don't get pregnant!), you should not be doing anything you don't enjoy (but don't get pregnant!), this is supposed to be about your pleasure, as well as his (but don't get pregnant!).

The hidden agenda behind this speech is to encourage young women to stop and think about why they are having sex. We are saying it's not something you should do just to keep a boyfriend, or to satisfy him. (I'm sorry, Orlando, if you don't particularly want to hear this from your mother, but medicine washes most of the modesty right out of doctors, placing our children in the position of being far more easily abashed than we are. Don't worry, you'll get there yourself; someday you'll find yourself embarrassing your teenager at the dinner table.)

I doubt that I solved Jeanette's dilemma, but I hope I left her feeling that she was fully entitled to take her time and make her choice—and that it was important she not get pregnant! I hope I made it clear that if and when she did decide it was time to be sexually active—when her body and her brain agreed—she could come to see me and get nonjudgmental medical assistance in staying healthy and not pregnant.

Orlando, whatever kind of medicine you choose, you will be in so many people's lives. You will know their secrets, and their family secrets. I knew what Jeanette's mother had thought about her when she was five, and when she was thirteen. I knew about some times when her mother had felt like giving up. I knew about her older son who was in jail. I knew about their family and their family struggles. Over the course of our years together, I had even worried a couple of times that her mother was just too stressed—she had two older boys who gave her a lot of trouble, she was often out of work, she had medical problems of her own—and I had seriously contemplated calling the department of social services to report that her children were at risk. I never did that—in part because I convinced myself that the mother was managing and that the kids were okay, in part because I was afraid that if I did it, my relationship with this family would be over.

This is the privilege of the profession: You get to be part of so many lives and so many stories. Sometimes I look through an old notebook and read my notes about someone I've forgotten—someone whose story was crowded out by all the other stories—and the image of that forgotten child comes back full force, and I can't believe it could ever have slipped my mind. Once, when I was about to go on vacation, I was winnowing my guilty pile of patient follow-up papers, trying to act on anything that looked time-sensitive. I came across a computer printout, a lab test result, and found myself wondering why this was even in my pile: a fully normal complete blood count on a two-year-old, Daniel Smith, from months ago. Daniel wasn't a child who needed to start taking iron drops. All the indices were normal; there was a proper number of normally sized and normally pigmented red blood cells. I couldn't have kept the paper on my desk to remind me to talk to a hematologist, because nothing looked out of whack. I should have long ago signed off on the numbers electronically. Why had I held on to the paper backup record? Had I kept the lab results in my pile only to remind myself that the child himself existed?

His name rang no particular bell; it was a common first name and a common surname. I looked at his blood count irritably. Why was I keeping normal test results? But at the same time I also worried that I had kept the paper in the pile as a way of reminding myself Daniel Smith needed follow-up for some other reason. I clicked my way into the medical record, clicked on his number, and waited for his chart to appear on the screen.

Then, in those microseconds while the computer called him up, I remembered who he was. He was the two-year-old who had died in a house fire. He was the two-year-old whose family had awakened smelling smoke, whose father had grabbed him and leaped with him out of an upper-story window. The father was injured, the son was killed in the fall. Other children in the family were badly hurt by smoke inhalation. And only a day or two before all this happened, my two-year-old patient's father had brought him in for a checkup, and as part of the checkup I had sent him to have his blood drawn. By the time the official printout came into my box, the child was dead, and I hadn't known what to do with the piece of paper. I should have initialed it and dropped it into the medical records box for filing. But I couldn't sign off on it, I couldn't let it disappear back into medical records, and I couldn't throw it away or shred it. It was like holding on to one last tiny thread linking me to this child, to the real, live, vigorous two-year-old who had let me listen to his heart and lungs and then protested loudly when I tried to look into his ears, who had regarded me with deep and profound suspicion from the safety of his father's arms, and whose suspicions I had justified completely by sending him off to the lab to have his blood drawn.

I had ordered the test because Daniel had been quite anemic in the past. At his eighteen-month visit, I had checked his hematocrit, a simpler, cheaper test requiring less blood and a routine test for children this age. Children are particularly vulnerable to iron-deficiency anemia from just before their first birthday to the age of two or three, especially those who are still getting much of their protein and other nutrition from milk.

So we check the blood count at nine months, and when it's low, I start the children on iron drops and talk to the parents about adding iron-rich foods to the child's diet. I say "start the children on iron drops" as if it were no sooner said than done. The fact is, it's a rare child who likes the taste of any of the available iron preparations, and a rare parent who is up to what is supposed to be a twice a day (or even three times a day) dosing schedule. Often the child comes back for the next visit and the hematocrit hasn't budged and the parent admits, sheepishly, that the iron has not been a regular daily feature.

Not this child. Daniel's father told me proudly at the checkup that he had given the iron drops faithfully, day in and day out. He had decreased the number of daily milk bottles and started letting the boy feed himself a variety of table foods. I sent him off for the more complete blood test, thinking he had now had a fair trial of iron, and I wanted to see his hematologic indices. They looked terrific. The iron drops had worked. He was no longer anemic. A tiny pediatric victory, a small step for parental commitment and consistency. The only thing was, by the time I got those encouraging lab results, the child was dead.

I held on to those lab results—and I'm still holding on to those lab results—because I couldn't bear to let them go. I held on to them, I guess, because they said something to me about the daily work and trouble of being a parent, of tending a two-year-old, about the ways love translates itself into detail and caretaking. I held on to those lab results because right after the child died, when I could still remember so clearly Daniel's alive, healthy two-year-old vigor in my exam room, I didn't want to let them go and see this last tiny medical link disappear.

So I put the paper on my pile, and then months went by as more children passed through the exam room and my memories faded. Whatever small, faint link I might have claimed disappeared into the mist—so much so that I blanked when I looked at the lab sheet and initially couldn't even remember the story that went with it.

This is a primary-care story, and a sad one. But here's a happier story, an account of obscure diagnosis and high-tech heroism. One day, right before the health center's Christmas party, I examined a two-week-old girl named Catriona whose mother was worried because she wasn't gaining weight. I ended up drawing labs, which showed that something was terribly wrong with Catriona's liver, so I sent her to the hospital. I remember I was wearing red crystal earrings that day because of the

Christmas party, and one fell out in the exam room, probably nudged out of place by my stethoscope earpiece, and Catriona's mother, terribly worried as she was, pointed this out and helped me find it.

At the hospital, Catriona was diagnosed with a rare genetic liver disease, alpha-1 antitrypsin deficiency, and she had one complication after another as her liver failed. I'm not sure anyone thought she would survive, but she got a liver transplant when she was two years old, and she did brilliantly. When I think about her, I remember that pasty, too-small baby in the exam room, and that desperately sick toddler in the intensive care unit when her liver was failing and her belly was swollen with fluid that shouldn't have been there. Then I think about her marching into the room for her five-year-old visit, a delightful child with a lot of well-healed scars on her belly.

I didn't save Catriona's life—the transplant surgeons did that, and above all the person who agreed to donate a child's liver after a terrible accident, and Catriona's parents, who hovered over her every hour of every day for months and months. I didn't save her life, but I was part of her life, and she was part of mine. When her family moved away and needed to change to a doctor in their new town, I missed them. Her photo hung on my bulletin board for years—a picture of Catriona with Mr. Rogers, someone she really loved. A charity that granted wishes for sick children had arranged for her to meet him, and every time I looked at the photo I would wonder what my role in her life was supposed to be. Should I be tracking her birthday, sending her a card every year? Should I call every once in a while: "Hi, this is your old pediatrician"?

I carry all these stories around with me—all doctors do. And I carry around the secrets. Every patient interview invites certain routine secrets: Tell me about substance abuse, about alcohol, about your sexual history. Those are some of the questions that medical students learn to ask, matter-of-factly, in those patient interviews I was talking about back at the beginning of the book. But how about my seventeen-year-old patient who had been raised by strict religious parents and felt terribly guilty that she was having sex with her boyfriend—so guilty that she couldn't admit it to herself, so she didn't use birth control. Her sex life was a secret from her parents, but when she got pregnant, she wanted to keep that secret from her boyfriend because she was afraid he would be angry. So the abortion was a secret from her parents *and* from her boyfriend—and so was the second abortion. I certainly didn't feel I was doing a very good job as her doctor—or she wouldn't have had those abortions—but I understood that part of my job was to help her carry her secrets.

Or the woman in her thirties with the newborn twins who told me in a whisper that yes, she had a much older son who had been born when she was only twenty. But that child had been taken away by the state, and please don't ever tell her husband. "I don't want him to know I used drugs so heavily," she said. "I don't want him to worry that I had a child taken away and I don't know how to take good care of children."

What do you do, as a doctor, with all the stories you hear and with all the secrets you know? I don't mean, exactly, what do you do—because you know what to do—you use the stories and the secrets to try to take proper care of your patients' medical problems, to answer the questions that bring them to you, to do your job. But how do you handle this knowledge, these secrets?

I'm talking about confidentiality. When I trained, we didn't think much about it. We knew medical information was supposed to be confidential, and there were sometimes signs in the hospital elevators reminding staff not to discuss patients in public places. We understood we weren't supposed to carry home tales of celebrity patients or tell stories out of the hospital using people's real names. But beyond that there were no particular rules and, I would have to say, no high level of consciousness. I had certainly never thought about the physical security of medical information, about who had access to medical records.

In 1996, Congress passed HIPAA—the Health Information Portability and Accountability Act. It protects employees' health insurance when they change jobs (that's the portability part) and it required new standards—and major changes—in the handling of health information. Now when you go see your doctor and you're asked to sign a document about where and how your health information can be released—that's HIPAA. When the health center gets inspected and there's a penalty for displaying a chart in the Plexiglas slot on an exam room in such a way that passersby can read the name—that's HIPAA. There are stiff penalties now for HIPAA violations—for giving medical information out to anyone who isn't entitled to it—and we all think much more carefully than we used to before we blab.

Is this always good? Clearly, as a patient you don't want your medical information leaking all over the place, and electronic records and databases had raised that risk. You don't want the airlines selling discount package tours to Las Vegas to have access to your therapy records in which you discuss your gambling problem. You don't want the guys who are marketing an expensive new antihypertensive drug to have access to the database where your blood pressure is tracked. HIPAA has forced us all, patients and medical professionals, to remember that. But it's also created a tremendous amount of paperwork (all those forms that everyone signs but no one reads), and sometimes it makes for great awkwardness in practice. I would see a patient who had been seen the day before in an emergency room, and I'd call the emergency room to find out what lab work had been done, and when I finally got through the emergency room switchboard—after listening to the canned music for a long time—someone would tell me, sorry, we can't give out any lab results until you fax us a signed release from the mother; no we can't take a verbal authorization. At that point I would want to say, for crying out loud, just what ulterior motive do you think I could have for wanting to know if a seven-year-old has strep throat? Instead, I would have to get the mother to sign a release form, fax it over, wait for it to go through, wait for someone to pick it up, and then start all over again with the switchboard, while the rest of my patients cooled their heels in the waiting room. The other day I listened to a colleague give a parent a child's lab results over the phone, and after he hung up, he looked at me and said, probably a HIPAA violation, don't report me.

You should take the imperative of confidentiality and discretion with great seriousness—and you should break the rules every now and then if that's what the patient needs to get good care. People's medical charts hold all kinds of information, and patients give doctors other information that we decide it is the better part of valor to keep out of the charts. For example, when that mother told me about having a child taken away in another state, I didn't put that in the newborn's medical record. I was afraid someone might see it and refer to it, maybe in front of her husband, so I told myself it belonged maybe in the mother's chart but not in this other baby's record.

By now you're probably wondering about those patient stories I've been telling. How can I rattle on about confidentiality and then tell these stories? Or did I make them up? Jeanette's name is not Jeanette, needless to say, and I have changed some details in her story. Also, this happened so many years ago that I'm confident she would not recognize herself—or be recognized by anyone else—as a seventeen-year-old. Catriona, on the other hand, is really named Catriona, and I've changed no details. I know this is okay because years ago, soon after her liver transplant, I decided to write about taking care of this child (it's unusual in primary care at a neighborhood health center to have a child get a liver transplant). I asked her mother's permission, since the child would be so easily identifiable, even though I would change her name. Her mother read the essay I wrote, and her one request was that I change the name back to Catriona. She was proud of her daughter, proud of her whole family and how they had come through this experience. She was involved with organ donation as a cause, she was telling her own story publicly, and she wanted her daughter some day to read about herself. I restored the real name.

As for the Daniel Smith story, all the details of the child's illness are correct, but I have changed his name and his ethnicity. I have also withheld certain details of his life and death, which might have made it a better, more moving story, because I worried they would make the family identifiable. Every other patient story in this book is told either with permission or with altered identifying details.

But I wanted to write about "Daniel Smith"—I want to write about them all. Writing about medicine and about my patients has been part of my life in this profession since the beginning—since medical school and my training began. I like to think it has helped me keep perspective, and I like to think it has made me a better doctor than I would otherwise have been. I do believe that writing about my patients has stretched my skills of imagination and empathy.

I write about medicine because people want to read about medicine. In your medical training, you will find yourself entering a world that many people see as closed, inaccessible, and full of fascinating life-and-death secrets. As my training took me further into this world, and as I learned its customs and its language, I found myself trying to explain them to the people on the outside.

I won't pretend I write about medicine in order to be a better doctor to my patients, or in order to educate and inform the nonmedical world. I write about medicine because the field is full of fascinating stories, and because things happen to me every day that I want to chew over and retell and think about and understand and bring to other people's attention. I write about medicine because medicine reminds me every day that the world is full of characters and stories and plots.

That is what I mean, in the end, when I pose the question, What do you do with these secrets and these stories? I write about patients because, in one way or another, they have changed my world. Watching Jeanette grow up and struggle and succeed taught me so much about not writing off adolescents who go through a difficult time. Stumbling through the liver transplant with Catriona and her family made me feel technically and medically helpless—they needed a donated liver and a transplant surgeon with a whole transplant team—but I learned so much about how families can hold together even in the harshest times. I tell their stories, often just for my own eyes so that I don't break confidentiality, because telling them to myself helps me understand them and understand myself.

Knowing secrets can sometimes feel like a burden, so you should find ways to learn from them and talk back to them. I've come home so many times with stories to tell—funny stories or upsetting stories, stories I want to tell and discuss so someone else will feel scandalized or worried. But I don't tell; I really do keep secrets. Even if your patients' stories feel like a weight, you should respect their power, take them seriously, protect them, and hold them close. They are part of your job description, part of your responsibility, and part of your reward.

## 9

## ■ Death and Dying and Presiding

*The patient is a twenty-three-year-old female with metastatic osteosarcoma, status/post multiple courses of chemotherapy and multiple surgeries. She is admitted now for comfort measures and has signed a Do Not Resuscitate order.*

*The patient is a eight-year-old boy who was running to catch a school bus when he was struck by a pickup truck traveling at approximately fifty miles an hour. He was thrown at least ten feet, landing on his head. He has suffered extensive facial bruising, closed head injury, fractures of both lower extremities and one wrist, and possible abdominal trauma, and he was found to be unresponsive at the scene. He was intubated by the EMTs and brought to the hospital, where he has remained in the intensive care unit, in a state of coma.*

*The patient is a three-month-old infant, born full-term to a thirty-year-old G1P0–1 female, pregnancy without complications, baby previously well, growing and developing normally, who presented to the emergency room with cough, fever, and progressive respiratory distress. Her chest x-ray revealed bilateral lung opacities, and she was admitted and started on antibiotics for a presumed bacterial pneumonia, but it has become increasingly difficult to keep her oxygen levels up, and she is now transferred to the intensive care unit. A repeat chest x-ray shows an increasingly interstitial pattern. . . .*

*Dear Orlando,*

Oh, my dear, I have been in at so many deaths. It comes with the territory, even in pediatrics. The first time a child died in my hands—under my hands—was in my residency, during a failed resuscitation attempt. I will not forget it: the feeling of pulling back my hands from her chest, where I had been doing the compressions, the knowledge that my hands could do no good, and the momentary despair, wondering what was the use of all this training if my hands couldn't do this little girl any good. She had died in a car accident, which reflects the reality of how children die in the United States at this time in history. The leading cause of death in children and adolescents is "unintentional injuries," largely connected to cars. The next two are cancer and homicide, which is both a sad statement about our society and also, in a certain sense, a fortunate reality. It's not that there are so many car accidents and cases of cancer and homicides; those risks are on top today because the big infections that used to kill tens of thousands of children are now preventable. Because those childhood infections are no longer sweeping through the population, we have the great luxury of practicing pediatrics without ever really getting used to death. If I had had to train through a diphtheria epidemic, or a measles epidemic, or a polio epidemic, pediatric death might feel different to me—not acceptable, but more inevitable, more recognizable.

In adult medicine, death is inevitable and recognizable. A death in an adult emergency room is a matter of course—an overwhelming heart attack or stroke, or a debilitated nursing home resident sent in with a terminal infection. But a death in a pediatric emergency room is always notable, always unexpected, always traumatic for all the doctors and nurses. A good and sensitive internist or family physician, as part of the job, expects to help at the end of many adult lives, and will be involved again and again in advising patients and families as they try to make sane and wise decisions about how far to push medical care. A good and sensitive pediatrician expects to see all the patients wave goodbye and move on into their adult lives, where their eventual decades-away deterioration and death will be the internist's responsibility. Adults often worry that at the end of their lives, when they are elderly and sick, they will get more aggressive medical attention than they want. They sign medical proxies and make living wills in part because they worry doctors will prolong their lives into some kind of intensive care unit purgatory. Those aren't questions that generally worry children—or their parents. A child doesn't need a medical proxy; the parent is the decision maker. But with children you tend to fight hard and throw on the medical interventions while there is any hope left at all.

So I think one reason I chose pediatrics was because you don't have to accept the death of many of your patients as inevitable. You can fight every battle—or almost every battle—as if it can be won, as if the child can and should survive and live to grow up. Even so, I have been in at so many deaths.

•

The first case, described above, was a young woman I didn't know well at all. When I was a medical student starting my first clinical rotation, internal medicine, she was in a room on the ward, dying. I heard about her briefly on morning rounds. There was nothing more anyone could do for her, and we medical students were told to leave her alone. She was dying: "comfort measures only." Her family needed to be with her, and they needed peace and quiet. The resident who led our team didn't want to hear any more than that; he wanted to hear about the patients who still presented medical problems, the patients we could diagnose or treat. Maybe he didn't want to hear about the dying twenty-three-year-old because she represented a therapeutic failure, or maybe he was just uncomfortable with the whole idea of death and dying and wanted to wall it off as completely as possible.

That wouldn't be at all surprising. It's often been charged that doctors aren't comfortable with dying patients, that we don't know how to behave around dying patients, that we tend to avoid them, that we fail to offer help or comfort. But as the evidence has accumulated that, in fact, doctors don't do a very good job with dying patients and their families, it's become more common for medical schools to address this directly by offering courses about death and dying and the care of the dying patient.

An interesting medical education article entitled "The last hours of living: practical advice for clinicians" has this to say:

> *Most clinicians have little or no formal training in managing the dying process or death. Many have neither watched someone die nor provided direct care during the last hours of life. Families usually have even less experience or knowledge about death and dying. Based on media dramatization and vivid imaginations, most people have developed an exaggerated sense of what dying and death are like.*

*However, with appropriate management, it is possible
to provide smooth passage and comfort for the patient
and all those who watch.*

The article details the physical changes leading up to death (weakness, respiratory difficulty, etc.). It also provides detailed descriptions of how you can determine that death has occurred, and it even offers guidelines for notifying family members (what do you say when you get someone on the phone?).

I didn't know any of this when I started my residency. As a medical student on the wards, I had been around plenty of deaths—I had seen codes happen, emergency resuscitations, and I had filled the traditional medical student role, running back and forth to the lab with tubes of blood. When that twenty-three-year-old woman died, I was aware of her large family gathering and grieving and more vaguely aware of the years and years of struggle with the disease represented by her thick hospital chart. But she wasn't my patient. It wasn't my job to keep her comfortable or break bad news to her family or pronounce her dead. Her death stands out in my mind because she was a woman close to my age, and so I was frightened and saddened by what had happened to her. She got through the protective wall I was trying to construct between all those sick hospitalized patients and me.

When I started my residency in the newborn intensive care unit, it was the nurses who taught me what to do at a death. When a baby was born too premature to resuscitate, the practice then was to let the baby's parents hold it until its heart had completely stopped. Today, the boundary of what is too small to resuscitate has been pushed further and further back; I don't know how premature you have to be these days to meet with this gentle, but mortal, fate. Back then, the nurses had developed a "death kit"—a Polaroid camera to photograph the baby so the parents could have some pictures, a birth certificate where the tiny footprint would be preserved, and a nice blanket the parents could wrap the baby in. My job, the nurses told me, would be to baptize the baby if the parents wanted the baby baptized and a priest couldn't be found in time. And they taught me how. Then, when the heart stopped, it was my job to "pronounce" the baby dead.

The nurses in the NICU knew much more about taking care of sick and premature babies than I did. They had clinical skill, they had experience. Yet technically, we residents were in charge. There were all kinds of tensions as NICU nurses "suggested" orders and medications to new interns, who felt they really should be the ones running the place. A smart intern quickly learned that your best bet for successfully getting through the night in the NICU—and more important, for successfully getting the babies through the night—was to do what the nurses said. So I learned how to baptize babies. After all, I was an intern; I was learning new skills every day. Most of those skills were about keeping people alive, but it was also clear that the nurses regarded certain aspects of death as the doctor's dominion. They would comfort the family and take care of the actual body, but there were official roles—baptizing the dying or pronouncing the moment of death—that were ritually turned over to the doctor.

In the midst of a terrible, tragic night, I would suddenly find myself taking pride in my arcane expertise. At least I know that the death certificate has to be signed in *blue* ink; I won't make the mistake of signing in black. I learned how to baptize a dying baby by baptizing a dying baby (the nurse had shown me how to sprinkle the water and whispered to me the line to recite); how to pronounce a patient dead by being called in the middle of the night to pronounce a patient dead (the nurse assured me the child was dead and whispered to me what I was supposed to do—check the pulse, check the heart, check the time, and pronounce); how to fill in a death certificate by filling in a death certificate (the nurse reminded me about using blue ink).

•

The eight-year-old in the second case was one of my regular patients at the health center. A colleague called and told me he'd been hit by a car and wasn't doing well, so I went to the intensive care unit and I sat with his family. I knew enough by then, some years into practice, to understand that sometimes all you can do is sit with the family. They understood the situation, and it didn't look good. The boy was not responding to speech, not responding to pain, not responding to anything. Not much brain activity. CT scans showed lots of swelling inside the brain. Vital signs were unstable. I thought of my own children, of course, Orlando, I thought of you. I thought about having a healthy, bright, active eight-year-old one day and the next day finding yourself at the beginning of a new lifetime full of sorrow and regret and might-have-beens. So I sat with them. I came back to sit some more the next day, and the next. Things didn't get better. I talked to the ICU doctors, who were beginning to conclude that things weren't going to get better. The family knew this, I think, knew it well before the painful meeting at which they were formally given the news, and at which they said, if his brain is gone, please turn off the machines.

The question of who delivers such news is delicate all by itself. There is a whole set of overlapping and sometimes contradictory traditions and practices here, and once again, it wasn't something that anyone ever taught us how to do. It makes sense to have bad news—the worst news—delivered by someone who really knows the patient, knows the family, and knows the medicine

involved, by someone with real experience and real authority. Unfortunately, sometimes each of those someones
is a different person, and sometimes all good intentions
go out the window because the news has to be delivered
and the only person around has to do it. In this case, the
person who led the meeting, appropriately enough, was
the PICU attending, who knew the medical situation inside and out. I was present as the person who knew the
family and had known the child well, and we did our best.
I suppose you could say we did it right, but under the circumstances, it's hard to know what that means.

You know who I envied most during this time? I envied their priest, who was also a daily visitor. I envied
him because it seemed to me that he offered them gen-
uine help and comfort. Death was a part of his job description, just as it was a part of mine, and it found him
prepared with comfort and ritual; he faced it with confidence. He knew what he was doing was the right thing
to do, and he believed it mattered. I, on the other hand,
was aware of my own uselessness, and the uselessness of
my whole profession, even the high-tech ICU. Medical
science was not saving this child and could not save this
child. I did what I could in my own particular role: I sat
with the family and we talked about the child, I tried to
help them understand the medical information they
were given, I identified the various doctors involved if
the parents had questions. But sometimes I had the distinct sense that the parents were trying hard to be kind

to me, to make me feel useful, to thank me for any trivial piece of information I provided. They would have been grateful for any medical help, but as it became clear that medicine could not help, they looked to their priest, and he had real help to offer, though of a different kind.

I asked to be present when the family was approached about organ donation. I didn't think they were going to consent, and in fact they didn't. A healthy child who is hit by a car is an excellent candidate for organ donation, and anyone who works in pediatrics knows how valuable those organs can be. My little patient with the alpha-1 antitrypsin deficiency is alive today because someone donated a liver. So yes, I had hoped this boy's parents would find some comfort in the idea of donating his organs, but I just didn't believe they would do it. The ICU resident asked this question—which was carefully not asked as part of the meeting where the decision to pull back on care was made—and he asked it well, carefully, respectfully, offering them some time to think about it. But they didn't want time to think about it; they wanted to say no. We don't want him cut up in any way, they said, we don't want to do this.

I think one reason I envied the priest was that death was a part of his job, but in no way did this child's death constitute a professional failure. I, on the other hand, experienced the death as a medical failure; a child had been brought to the hospital to recieve help and the "help" had not been enough.

•

The third vignette is also about unhappy outcomes and death—and about breaking bad news—but it's also about some of the living you do in the shadow of death. Mary was three months old when she was admitted to the hospital with pneumonia, respiratory distress, and hypoxia (low oxygen). This was sixteen years ago, when I was a fellow doing my pediatric infectious diseases training, and back then those symptoms made us worry about AIDS. This clinical pattern—respiratory distress, hypoxia, the classic interstitial pattern on the chest x-ray showing disease in between the air sacs—is strongly suggestive of pneumocystis pneumonia, which often signaled the initial appearance of HIV disease in young children. It was bad news any way you looked at it—bad news because it made you worry that the child was infected with HIV, and bad news because it was an opportunistic infection, which meant the virus had already knocked out the child's immune system and left her incredibly vulnerable. If she had pneumocystis, she didn't just have HIV, she had AIDS. And it was bad news because pneumocystis pneumonia was a dangerous infection, especially in a young infant.

It was my job to tell Mary's parents what we were worried about and to ask their permission to test for HIV. We didn't test the baby, who was too young to be making antibodies to the virus; instead we tested her mother. After all, if Mary did have HIV—if her illness was indeed an opportunistic infection attacking her because her immune system was damaged by the virus—then she had congenital HIV; her mother was infected. The test was positive. It was my job to deliver this result to the family. I would have to tell the mother she was infected with HIV, and then we would have to deal with the question of whether her husband was also infected, which might have all kinds of ramifications in their marriage. I would have to advise her husband to get tested. I would have to tell them both that the baby was infected. I would have to tell the mother that the disease had already progressed to the point where her daughter had little immune system left. In other words, it was my job to destroy this mother's life—or that was how it felt to me.

The parents took this news in the best spirit possible—they chose to focus on the baby and her health, and they seemed to be able to support one another. The mother cried, the father comforted her, and I found myself retreating, as doctors often do, into medical details: We'll treat her with this and we'll test her for that and when she's better we'll add this medication and we'll see her regularly in our clinic.

But at least we were successful in treating Mary. In fact, we had been so sure she had pneumocystis that we had started treating her before the HIV results came back. Her oxygenation improved, and she got better and went home and then started coming to the pediatric HIV clinic, which had a large team of doctors and nurses and social workers and nutritionists. But I stayed involved as her primary infectious diseases doctor. I saw her whenever she came to the clinic, I stayed in touch with the family, and I thought of myself as the person who knew her best, from a medical point of view. Over the course of the next year, I saw her over and over again, and I got to know her well. We tried to get her to grow and gain weight, and we tried to rebuild her immune system. I probably don't have to tell you this, but she was a beautiful baby, and when she felt well she would smile and coo and babble. Of course, I'm just telling you that to make you cry. Yes, she was a beautiful baby, but this would have been just as sad a story if she hadn't been.

Mary is one of those children who would probably do well today. She might have a better chance from the start, because her mother would most likely have been tested for HIV during pregnancy—the test is supposed to be offered to all pregnant women; it's not compulsory, but it is recommended. If the mother had known she was positive, she could have taken medications that would have greatly reduced the odds of passing on the virus to her baby. But we didn't know how to do any of this back then. If she hadn't been tested, and Mary had still ended up HIV-positive, we have better antiretroviral drugs to offer, and she would have had a fighting chance to grow up. So I could be telling you this story as one of my tales of science and progress and the strange sense of regret that comes when you look at patients who were just a little too early for the miracles that we're so proud of in medicine. It's hard to predict which miracles the next ten years will hold, but I'm sure that if I worked with children who had cancer, for example, I would feel a particular agony every time a child died of a disease for which new treatments seem tantalizingly close. That's why you enroll patients in clinical trials, after all, hoping always to crowd them in, over that borderline, into the treatments of tomorrow.

That's not why I'm telling you Mary's story. I'm telling you because the story ended with Mary's funeral, about a year after her diagnosis. I'm telling you her story because it was the first time I'd known a patient this well, known a family this well. I found myself at the funeral, with nothing left to do but cry.

I know it sounds strange, Orlando, but if you are fortunate in your medical career, you will attend a few funerals. I say "fortunate," because attending will reflect your deep involvement with certain families, involvement that extends past the reach of what medical science can do. In fact, sometimes you may be at a funeral to bear witness to medical failure. Sometimes you will be there because you have come to care about a family, and you know they have come to care about you, and you know that your presence will be meaningful to them. Going to a funeral—like sitting with that eight-year-old boy's family—is something you can do when you can't do anything else. It's part of being on terms with death, and in our job you have to be on terms with death. You have to understand that death is sometimes the enemy to be fought or evaded, and that death is sometimes inevitable and sometimes even welcome. But it's not something that you can turn away from or ignore. You need to know the science and the technicalities, the forms and the legalities, the rites and the rituals. None of us will ever completely understand death, just as medicine will never succeed in conquering it, but we can look closely at both the weaknesses of human bodies and the surpassing strengths of the spirit, the heart, and the intellect. It's in your job description and it's part of your job, as I said to you about stories and secrets. That's because death is eventually part of everyone's story and part of the great secret that draws us all into medicine.

# 10

## ■ Work and Life

*The patient is a fifty-five-year-old woman with severe inflammatory bowel disease, and you have been her primary-care physician for over a decade. She is highly anxious, and though you have, among other interventions, prescribed antianxiety medication, she continues to manifest a high degree of anxiety, especially about medical catastrophes and the possibility of dying. She has told you repeatedly that you are the only doctor she really trusts. In recent years, her GI symptoms have been reasonably well controlled, but she remains terrified with each new flare of her chronic disease. You are in the car with your family, heading to the airport for a well-earned vacation, when your beeper goes off. This patient is in the emergency room with severe abdominal pain and a significant GI bleed. Although she knows you are not on call, she requested that you be paged and informed of her condition.*

*Dear Orlando,*

We come at last to what kind of life you are going to build around your work, and the work that will be your life. I want to talk to you about taking care of your patients, about taking care of yourself and your family, and maybe a little about taking care of the world.

Let's start with your patients. When I was a second-year medical student, I took a course called Introduction to Clinical Medicine. You'll recall that this is where we learned to do physical exams—first on one another, then on patients—and to interview patients and take their histories. This was the course that was supposed to guide our transition from classroom-sitting lecture-going test-taking fact memorizers into patient-touching history-taking junior physicians. For the first time in our medical school careers, we were regularly reporting to a hospital, self-conscious in our short white coats, starting to stuff the pockets with devices—the otoscope to check people's ears, the tuning fork to assess conductive hearing, the reflex hammer. We slung our stethoscopes around our necks and tried to wear them as if we felt entitled to them. We also carried an assortment of small published manuals that promised to provide all the essential information we would ever need. Some of these had serious titles like *Essential Digest of Clinical Internal Medicine;* others, less formal, made embarrassing claims: *The Medical Student's Practical Guide to Surviving Your Clinical Rotations,* or *The Scut Handbook.* You could weigh down the pockets of that short white coat as you waddled through the hospital halls: a manual on either side, covers carefully positioned so that no one would see you were carrying around a book called *The Complete Scut-Puppy,* the tuning fork and otoscope clanking against each other in your breast pocket. Occasionally, helpfully, a resident or an attending would remind you of the hospital truism, full pockets, empty mind.

This period in my medical education felt like an important transitional moment, weighted in more ways than my pockets. Here I was finding my way around the hospital with increasing confidence, clutching my tools and my crib sheets and my guidebooks, interviewing and examining patients, learning, finally, from real practicing physicians. In the first two years of medical school, many of our professors had been basic scientists—anatomists, physiologists, biochemists, cell biologists, geneticists. Sure, they brought in physicians to do some of the lectures, and sure, some of those physicians talked about their patients—or even brought them in to appear before the whole class for the occasional clinical correlations session—but this was different. In Introduction to Clinical Medicine, the dignified white-coated professors were serious physicians, on their own ground, in their own kingdom. They wore long white coats, without bulging pockets (empty pockets, full mind, the residents reminded us), and they knew how to use their stethoscopes. They held the keys.

The doctor in charge of our course would meet with us regularly and present us with patient scenarios. By this point I was used to these scenarios; I had encountered them in course after course, I was accustomed to seeing them on problem sets or tests. But again, this was different—he was using stories from his own experience, and he was using them to make teaching points about doctoring in general, rather than specific diseases. His job, after all, was to teach us to be doctors.

One day he presented a version of the case I described, the long-term patient who comes to the emergency room terrified and asking to see you, as the beeper is going off on your way to the airport. What would you do, he asked? Stay in the cab, keep going to the airport? Abandon your family, rush to the emergency room? Were there any other alternatives? What did professionalism require, what did compassion dictate?

I still remember the embarrassed hush that came over our small group of medical students. What was the right answer? What if you said, "I would immediately rush to the emergency room to take care of my patient"? Would you look like a goody-goody? Would the course director gently but firmly explain that doctors also needed to protect their private lives and their families, and that the important thing was to have systems in place to make sure the patient was getting good care? Or if you offered an answer about staying with your family, because, after all, your family needed you too, would he shake his head and explain that the physician's first obligation was to the patient? I had never heard anyone pose such a question before, and I found myself immediately pulled in both directions. I could imagine the way my family would react if I diverted the long-planned, well-deserved vacation. But I could also imagine that patient, whom I had been treating for ten years, asking for me in the emergency room. Would my professional ethic be compromised if I let her down? Or would the director smile and point out that I might have hundreds of such patients, and how could I change my vacations or my other plans every time one of them had an emergency?

Like any medical student, what I really wanted was to get the right answer and impress my teacher and my fellow students. But I knew that getting the right answer to this particular question was more subtle and complicated than being the first to pop up with the definition of a pulsus paradoxus or a precordial gallop. This was a question about real life, and I didn't know the answer.

In the meantime, there was that anxious woman in the emergency room, bleeding into her gut. Hesitantly, we medical students began to offer answers. Even though we were experienced at answering questions, we could see the traps looming ahead. Someone suggested, maybe I could call a colleague and ask my colleague to go check on her. Another person said, I think I would ask to speak to her and see how she was doing. Someone else said, maybe if I go to the emergency room and see her and explain the situation. Finally, the professor entered the discussion. Yes, he said, you might be able to find someone else who could cover, especially if you've thought it through in advance and built up those relationships. Yes, you might be able to speak to the patient on the phone and make her feel you are supervising her care, that you agree with what her doctors are doing, that you know the people caring for her and think they're doing the right thing, that you're sending a colleague to see her. Or yes, you might interrupt your trip to the airport, or even send your family ahead on vacation and plan to catch up with them. The point I am trying to make, he said, is that this is a serious question. You have to think about it; you have to do something. It is part of your responsibility and part of your identity. You do not get to shrug and say, hey, I'm not on call; you do not get to say that this is not your problem. She is your patient, and it is your problem. You are this woman's physician, you have built a relationship, and she trusts you, and what she trusts you with is what she considers life and death. How you handle this question will reflect your professional standards and your practice and who you are.

I'm not sure those were his exact words. But I remember exactly how I felt as I listened to him. I knew what he was saying would reverberate for all of us as we moved through our lives. No one had ever said anything like this to us before, something at once deeply personal and profoundly professional. I suppose we felt that in even asking the question, he was acknowledging that we were close to becoming real doctors. I have thought of it so many times over the past twenty years that I'm no longer sure how much is paraphrase of my professor's statement and how much is my own voice, looking at my own life.

Orlando, how much of a sense did you have that my professional life sometimes intruded into our family life? Do you remember me on vacations, obsessed with placing an international phone call so I could double-check some patient's lab result or so I could ask a colleague whether a sick child had recovered? I remember standing at a public phone in one of the world's great museums—the Louvre? the Vatican?—and urging a mother in Dorchester, Massachusetts, to bring her little girl in for a repeat urine test, because I had already called a colleague to find out the results, and my colleague had told me the mother had missed the follow-up appointment. I'm not offering you this image as proof of my remarkable dedication. I'm telling you that when you really feel you're someone's doctor, you can't take yourself out of the story on a technicality. You think about what the patient needs and, as the professor told us all those years ago, you think about what it will take to get the patient cared for. You don't necessarily have to do it all yourself. That's why he emphasized planning your cross-coverage properly and trusting your colleagues. I would also emphasize how important it is to moderate your own anxiety levels. If you spend your whole vacation double-checking every normal lab result and second-guessing the people who are covering you, the problem is probably with your own internal settings.

In my first letter, I told you why there was a special sweetness for me, as a woman, a woman doctor, a woman doctor of my generation, in your decision to go to medical school. I haven't spent my professional life worrying that my career in medicine was shortchanging you and your brother and sister. On the other hand, I've always known that medicine pulls hard—famously harder than any other profession, at least at the training stage—and I've often felt pulled. I like the idea that you find this combination of life and work appealing. But as you know, it's not been exactly easy in our family.

Do you remember me arguing with your father? The worst fights happened when I was doing my residency and fellowship and my hours were so unpredictable. I would promise to pick you up from day care, and I would be sure that I would be out in plenty of time. Then something would come up, and I would find myself calling your father and saying, "I don't think I'll make it after all. Can you pick him up, please? Thank you. Sorry." Sometimes he was cheerful and generous about it, and sometimes he was grouchy and irritated. He was entitled to be, I guess. I was always breaking my promises.

Maybe if I were a trauma surgeon, my promise breaking would at least have had the drama of life and death: "I'm sorry, I can't pick up our son at day care because there's been a ten-car accident on the interstate, and they're bringing in six patients by ambulance and two patients by helicopter—gotta run now, honey, talk to you later, when I've saved a few lives." But what I do is rarely so dramatic. I'm usually staying late because an eight-year-old boy had a bad asthma attack and I sent him to the emergency room by ambulance and things got backed up. Or because I spent an hour trying to track down a specialist to ask a question about a teenager with an odd rash, and when I finally reached the specialist and described the rash, he thought it sounded like an unusual vasculitis and suggested I do a bunch of labs to look for autoimmune disorders, and I'm waiting for results to come back. Or because a teenager came in to be checked for swimmer's ear and revealed that her father was abusing her, and we're still sorting out where she's going to go from here, since she can't go home. Some event of this magnitude will reliably occur every couple of days in primary care. This is what makes me reliably unreliable in the service of checking lab results and re-turning phone calls—not performing heroic surgery.

Here's something I'm sure you don't remember: As a baby, you were not a good sleeper. When you were one, one and a half, two, you were perfectly willing to go to bed—you would get into your fuzzy pajamas with the feet, you would listen to *Goodnight, Moon*, you would be kissed and hugged, and you would go in your crib. In the middle of the night, you would wake up and discover yourself alone in the dark, and you would howl for company. As soon as someone appeared to reassure you, you would settle down and go back to sleep. Sometimes this happened once a night, sometimes twice.

During this period I was a third-year medical student, then an intern, then a resident, working more than one hundred hours a week (you remember how we calculated that). Unlike other hardworking mothers who usually make it home most nights, as a doctor-in-training I was at the hospital one night out of every three or four. Not surprisingly, your father felt that on the nights I was home, I ought to take my turn getting up to soothe you. So when you cried I would struggle to wake up from what seemed like the deepest, darkest sleep ever—the sleep of someone who has lived with that nervous on-call in-hospital sleep, and who is grateful to come home and shut out the world and sleep for real. If I was sleeping too deeply to hear you crying, your father would elbow me—hey, he's crying, it's your turn. Filled with exhaustion-tinged resentment, I would shuffle into your room, pat your fuzzy back, talk you into going back to sleep, then shuffle back to my own bed.

Quite a bit of resentment was going on then, all of it justified. I usually had to be at work too early to help in the morning, I often stayed too late to pick you up, I was gone for those on-call evenings and nights, I worked most weekends, and when I did come home I was so tired that I couldn't sit down without falling asleep. And I was so jealous of the time your father had with you, and of what seemed to me the limitless luxury of all those daylight hours outside the hospital and all those night-time hours of sleep, with only you to interrupt occasionally. Trust me, there was a certain amount of resentment on both sides.

Your father and I discussed the possibility of letting you cry at night to break the waking-up habit, but we agreed we were all too stressed right then to look for more battles. If you wanted company at night, we would go on reassuring you until you grew out of it.

And you did grow out of it. When you were in college and would come home on break and sleep until two p.m., your father and I would ruefully remind each other, Remember when he wasn't a good sleeper? I look back now to when you were waking up at night and Larry and I were resenting each other, and I remember how much my job was pulling on all of us, making it hard to see straight, making it hard to know what was fair and what was not. My job was echoing through our young family in all kinds of ways. At the same time, my job was a good job, and I was glad to be doing it.

Remember that I told you medical training will transform you. Medicine selects for people like us: competitive, mildly obsessive, conscientious, willing to work hard but sometimes addicted to that feeling of working harder than anyone else. It rewards us for obsessive work habits, it nourishes our anxieties about mistakes and responsibility, it offers us constant reminders that no matter how hard we try, we can never know everything, never keep up completely with the pace of new information.

Keep an eye out for what medicine does to you, Orlando, and to the people you love. Your patients will have a real claim on you—on your time, on your thoughts, on your behavior. Make the effort to imagine and understand their lives, to put yourself in the patient's place. Don't wall yourself off, and don't fool yourself into thinking that affections and emotions are somehow unprofessional. And be sure to value the people who help you and support you. When family, friends, even parents, put up with some inconvenience or some stress or some craziness because of your training and your schedule and your job and your patients, well, the right thing to say is thank you. Make sure you exercise your growing powers of empathy on the people around you. Look at the ones you love with the same attention and care and compassion that you expend on complex patients and differential diagnoses. And don't forget to say thank you.

I hope you won't let the pressures of your training drive out your other interests and passions. I got through medical training in part because I was able to write about it; I needed something in my life that used other parts of my brain, that awakened different senses, and that offered me a way to understand what was happening to me. Medical training changed me a lot; writing helped me to stay the person I am. Think about what you need to have in your life to stay the person you are while you're becoming the doctor you want to be. It's not easy to keep up your other interests and passions during your training, but it can be done. I did my residency with a dancer, and he kept dancing while he trained. I went to medical school with people who sang in the church choir and people who climbed cliffs. They couldn't do these things as regularly as they wanted to, but they didn't let go (well, cliff climbers aren't supposed to let go).

Finally, my dear, if you find along the way that you have a cause, an obsession, a way to change the world, give in to it and accept it as a gift. Many physicians find they want to contribute to big changes that go way beyond caring for individual patients. I have that recurring fantasy about spending time overseas sometime down the road—in refugee camps, in war zones. I don't think it's totally altruistic, either. When I visited Mother Theresa's House of Healing in Calcutta a couple of years ago, I met an Australian emergency room doctor. He was there on a religious medical mission to help the poor and the dying—but he was also so thrilled by the cases he was getting to see, the pathology, the diseases he'd only read about. I understand both sides of that, and so will you.

As you know, even before I have gotten to that when-the-children-are-grown stage, my professional life has been caught up in a cause. More than a decade ago, I got involved with a pediatric literacy organization called Reach Out and Read and have been working since then with pediatricians and family physicians and nurse-practitioners and nurses to include children's books in primary-care visits. I believe everyone who takes care of young children should be advising parents that it's important to read to children, starting when they're babies, and I try to teach people how to work this into their everyday practice. Through Reach Out and Read, we give a free children's book at every checkup from six months to five years, which is ten books in the home by kindergarten.

Reach Out and Read is about early literacy—very early literacy. Consider how we learn spoken language; learning to talk doesn't start when you say your first words. If a baby doesn't hear language, if a baby doesn't practice by babbling, speech won't happen. Literacy—written language—doesn't start with learning to decode words in school. Children need to grow up handling books and hearing stories, they need the language exposure and the book exposure and the positive connections to books that are formed when parents and grandparents and other family members read to them. If they grow up without that, they arrive at school missing hours and hours of early literacy preparation.

Teachers will say they can tell on the first day of school which children have grown up without books. They know that children who grow up in poverty are at great risk for language problems: They are less likely to be read to, they are exposed to much less conversation, and they are at higher risk of falling behind in reading when they get to school. School success depends heavily on learning to read, and on learning to read on schedule, so that you go through school reading on grade level, and not below it. Parents need this message, especially parents living in poverty, and children need the books. By getting books into the hands of babies and toddlers and preschoolers through the people who deliver health care to them, we also link books to other essential aspects of children's health—to safety, to nutrition, to development—and we can offer guidance to parents and these books to their children in the first years of life.

Reach Out and Read has grown from a single program in a single hospital to a national program involving thousands of clinics and health centers and hospitals and practices. The program delivers advice and books to (as I write this) almost three million children every year, which is more than nine and a half thousand every day, most of them children growing up in poverty. Reach Out and Read has changed the practice of pediatrics. Doctors have been very enthusiastic. A great deal of what I do involves talking to them about how they can incorporate this into their practice without slowing down their pace, how they can use the books in the exam room to assess a child's fine-motor development, to ask about language—all things that pediatricians do routinely at every checkup. Doctors also embrace the program because they are persuaded by the evidence that it works. Studies published in the medical literature show that when doctors follow the Reach Out and Read model, parents read to their children more often, parents report more positive attitudes toward books and reading aloud, and starting at eighteen months, there are significant improvements in children's language skills.

I know I'm getting carried away. That's what happens when you find a cause, a way to save the world. But I believe, Orlando, that if every child grew up with books around, with the connection to books that comes from spending time as an infant and a toddler on a parent's lap, that it would go a little way to balance out some of the inequities that send so many of my patients to school completely unprepared, so set up for failure. I believe that the better a child's chance of succeeding in school and meeting with praise and reinforcement there, the better that child's chance of staying in school and getting to make real choices in life, rather than getting stuck in poverty and repeating parental patterns. I also believe that when we give books to parents, we're offering them a way to spend time with their children in a way that is positive and entertaining and rich in language, that we're helping put something into their daily life that is often missing in these times of electronic entertainment and the high stress levels with which many families function.

Yes, I've come full circle. I've talked us around to families and stress. As I have been saying, I want you to take care of your family, I want you to take care of yourself, but if you find your cause, I want you to be ready to take it up. Medicine attracts people who want to help, and sometimes wanting to help leads to wanting to change the world. I've met so many doctors who have found themselves caught up—often unexpectedly—in a quest to make changes, in advocacy, in policy, or just in some particular place. There are new trends in medicine—fixing the health care system, preventing medical errors, promoting the use of the medical apology—that have attracted physicians who combine academic interest with a zeal to make change happen. There's the pediatrician who retired from a suburban practice in Massachusetts and found herself more and more involved with Cambodian orphans—with building orphanages, with education, and with health care in Cambodia. There's the ob-gyn who goes regularly to Africa to repair vaginal fistulas and other childbirth-related injuries in women who would otherwise have their lives blighted.

So if you find your cause, make room for it in your already crowded life. Your life will surely be crowded, but you will get to choose all the different elements that cause the crowding. Your life will be crowded with skills, I hope, and with meaning and connections—and stories. Imagine yourself as a high-tech interventional cardiologist passing catheters into people's blood vessels. Imagine yourself as a primary-care internist with a busy waiting room. Imagine yourself doing eye surgery, or urological surgery, or heart surgery. Imagine yourself delivering babies, or taking care of sick babies in a newborn intensive care unit. Imagine yourself teaching medical students and passing along what you know. Even imagine yourself writing about your patients, or finding other ways to distill the lessons and the experiences and the stories that you hear to help other people understand. Find something that works for you—a place where you belong—and do the job properly. Take good care of your patients, take good care of the people you love, and take good care of yourself.

What an excellent, complicated, interesting job you've chosen. I believe you will do it well and honorably, which will mean a good and complicated and interesting life for you, and great comfort and healing for the many people whose lives you will touch. This is a privileged profession, and the greatest privilege of all is to have that contact with other lives, that opportunity to figure in so many people's stories, that chance to teach and learn and help and heal.

# Acknowledgments

When I was asked to write "letters to a young doctor," I immediately felt like something of an old—or at least aging—doctor. I sat down to write those letters and waited for the advice and wisdom to issue forth—and soon I felt like a less-than-wise old doctor. But I have been very lucky since the beginning of this project to have the advice and vision of my editor, Jo Ann Miller, who has helped tremendously in shaping this book, in sorting out its tone and its subject matter. I am also grateful to Elaine Markson for setting up and encouraging the project, and again, for her always sensible help and guidance.

My next set of acknowledgments starts in the clinic: I am deeply grateful to all the patients who have taught me, starting back in medical school and continuing right through last week: the families who have trusted me with their children, the parents who have told me their stories, the children who have puzzled me and worried me and gotten better with or without my help.

## Acknowledgments

I have been very fortunate in my professional life in finding myself among teachers and colleagues who have guided me and helped me not only to learn medicine, but to understand the pleasures and challenges of caring for patients. At Boston Medical Center, I was privileged to study with Doctors Jerome Klein and Stephen Pelton in Pediatric Infectious Diseases and to work for many years under the guidance of Doctor Barry Zuckerman.

I thank my colleagues at Boston Medical Center, Dorchester House, and New York University School of Medicine for all they have taught me about practicing medicine, and I want to mention in particular Holly Goodale and Emily Feinberg, with whom I saw patients every Tuesday evening for many years, and who were always ready to help me do better by my patients.

More recently, I have been lucky to find myself in the Department of Pediatrics at New York University, and I thank my new colleagues, especially Doctors Michael Weitzman, Benard Dreyer, and Arthur Fierman for making me welcome in the department and in a new clinical setting. I am also grateful to Doctors Lori Legano, Stephen Maddox, and Herbert Lazarus for the continuing education of working together, and to the many residents and medical students who have helped me think about the process of becoming a doctor.

Eileen Costello and Elizabeth Barnett have been the friends and colleagues with whom I discussed my most complicated, frightening, or frustrating medical conundrums ever since we completed residency, and I know I can still call them up, day or night, and say, without preamble, "Can I tell you about a kid?" Mitch Katz very kindly read the complete manuscript, offered many helpful suggestions, and reminded me to include the occasional adult patient. I acknowledge with gratitude the guidance of all who read this book in manuscript; many of the best thoughts and examples were suggested to me by these friends and colleagues. Of course, I am fully and completely responsible for any errors.

Then there's my family. I thank my parents, Morton and Sheila Klass, for supporting me through medical school, residency, and every other phase of my life. I know that my father, who died in 2001, would have enjoyed watching his first grandchild go to medical school—and he would probably have been the very first to credit Orlando with extensive medical knowledge and ask his advice. I will try—as I am always resolving to try—to support my children on their adventures through life with the same whole-hearted enthusiasm.

On the home front, Larry Wolff cheered me on through the writing of this book and read every page, offering helpful guidance and saving me from myself when I waxed too pompous. Anatol, our youngest child, sweetly put up with my absorption while I wrote the book and, at the age of eleven, naturally served as chief technical and Internet consultant (he is also the only one in the family who can make things print). Josephine, our college-student daughter, read the manuscript through and offered honest, detailed, and occasionally caustic comments. I enjoyed watching her keen critical intelligence at work. Finally, I thank my son, Benjamin Orlando Klass, for allowing me to write these letters to him, for allowing me once again to go public with stories about his birth and upbringing and now about his decision to go into medicine. Perhaps I should thank him as well, or at least congratulate him, for making that decision to go into medicine—but I've got the whole book in which to do that! I thank him also for reading the manuscript and making many helpful comments, and I tell him here once again that I am delighted to look forward to having him as a professional colleague.

## Selected References

Specific studies cited and comprehensive reports and summaries with extensive references on complex issues.

## Chapter 4

### *Resident work hours and the Libby Zion case*

Gaba, G. M., and S. K Howard. Fatigue among clinicians and the safety of patients. *New England Journal of Medicine* 2002; 347:1249–1255.

Robins, N. S. *The girl who died twice: every patient's nightmare: the Libby Zion case and the hidden hazards of hospitals.* New York: Delacorte Press, 1995.

## Chapter 5

### *Vaccines and autism*

Immunization Safety Review Committee. *Immunization safety review: vaccines and autism.* Washington, DC: National Academies Press, 2004.

## *Pulmonary artery catheters and patient mortality*

Connors, A. F., T. Speroff, N. V. Dawson, et al. The effectiveness of right heart catheterization in the initial care of critically ill patients. *JAMA* 1996;276:889–897.

Dalen, J. E., and R. C. Bone. Is it time to pull the pulmonary artery catheter? *JAMA* 1996;276:916–918.

## *Risk of severe bacterial infections in young children*

Mintegi, S., J. Benito, M. Gonzalez, E. Astobiza, J. Sanchez, and M. Santiago. Impact of the pneumococcal conjugate vaccine in the management of highly febrile children aged 6 to 24 months in an emergency department. *Pediatric Emergency Care* 2006 Aug;22(8):566–569.

Sard, B., M. C. Bailey, and R. Vinci. An analysis of pediatric blood cultures in the postpneumococcal conjugate vaccine era in a community hospital emergency department. *Pediatric Emergency Care* 2006 May; 22(5):295–300

Madsen, K. A., J. E. Bennett, and S. M. Downs. The role of parental preferences in the management of fever without source among 3- to 36-month-old children: a decision analysis. *Pediatrics* 2006 April; 117(4):1067–1076.

Isaacs, D., and D. Fitzgerald. Seven alternatives to evidence based medicine. *British Medical Journal* 1999; 1618–1618.

# Chapter 6

## *Doctors as patients*

Altman, L. K. The doctor's world; the man on the table was 97, but he devised the surgery. *The New York Times* December 25, 2006.

# Chapter 7

## *Medical Mistakes*

Institute of Medicine. *To err is human: building a safer health system.* Washington, DC: National Academies Press, 1999.

Leape, L. L., and D. M. Berwick. Five years after *To err is human*: what have we learned? *JAMA* 2005; 293:2384–2390.

Institute of Medicine. *Preventing medication errors.* Washington, DC: National Academies Press; 2006.

Ghaleb, M. A., N. Barber, B. D. Franklin, V. W. Yeung, Z. F. Khaki, and I. C. Wong. Systematic review of medication errors in pediatric patients. *Annals of Pharmacotherapy* 2006 October;40(10):1766–1776.

Gruen, R. L., G. J. Jurkovich, L. K. McIntyre, H. M. Foy, and R. V. Maier. Patterns of errors contributing to trauma mortality: lessons learned from 2,594 deaths. *Annals of Surgery* 2006 Sep;244(3):371–380.

Leape, L. L. Full disclosure and apology—an idea whose time has come. *Physician Executive* 2006; March–April:16–18.

Kilpatrick, K. Apology marks new era in response to medical error, hospital says. *Canadian Medical Association Journal* 2003;168 (6): 757.

# Chapter 9

### *Caring for dying patients*

Emanuel, L., F. D. Ferris, C. F. von Gunten, and J. H. Von Roenn. The last hours of living: practical advice for clinicians. CME article on Medscape (http://www.medscape.com/viewarticle/542262) "This text has been excerpted and adapted from: Emanuel, L., F. D. Ferris, C. F. von Gunten, and J. Von Roenn, editors. EPEC-O: Education in Palliative and End-of-life Care for Oncology. (Module 6: Last Hours of Living, The EPEC Project, Chicago, IL, 2005.)"

# Chapter 10

### *Reach Out and Read*

Mendelsohn, A. L., L. N. Mogilner, B. P. Dreyer, et al. The impact of a clinic-based literacy intervention on language development in inner-city preschool children. *Pediatrics* 2001;107:130–134.

Weitzman, C. C., L. Roy, T. Walls, and R. Tomlin. More evidence for Reach Out and Read: a home-based study. *Pediatrics* 2004;113;1248–1253.

High, P. C., L. LaGasse, S. Becker, I. Ahlgren, and A. Gardner. Literacy promotion in primary care pediatrics: can we make a difference? *Pediatrics* 2000;105: 927–934.

Klass, P. Pediatrics by the book: pediatricians and literacy promotion. *Pediatrics* 2002;110:989–995.